Worried Sick

CHAPTER 1

Introduction

WHAT IS STRESS?

- Naomi, a fifty-nine-year-old mother of five grown children, spent ten difficult years caring for her husband, Raymond, who was slowly dying from chronic liver disease. At the same time, Naomi worried about her mother, Marguerite, who was in the final stages of congestive heart failure and dementia. Just months after Ray and Marguerite died, Naomi suffered a transient ischemic attack (TIA) or "mini-stroke."
- Rob, a forty-seven-year-old copy machine repairman, was one of millions of Americans who lost his job during the recent recession. He went back to school for an associate's degree in computer science, developed new skills, and searched high and low for a new job—to no avail. After more than a year of fruitless job hunting, Rob shot and killed himself, leaving behind his devastated wife and teenage daughter.
- Marisol is a twenty-year-old dynamo who attends college full time, volunteers as a translator at her local hospital, works thirty-five hours each week at a fast-food restaurant to earn tuition money, and helps her single mother care for two younger sisters. An A- student majoring in

Spanish and biology, Marisol was so run down by the end of the semester that she fell sick with the flu, and had to take incompletes in two of her courses. She is worried that her grades may suffer, and that she won't be accepted into medical school.

We all know a Naomi, Rob, or Marisol. Each of us has witnessed a friend, coworker, or family member who tried to "do it all," yet ended up exhausted, sick, or depressed. Maybe you've faced your own struggles, whether a divorce, a bankruptcy, or a troubled relationship that pushed you to drink more than you usually would. Maybe you have a stressful job, and try to calm your nerves by smoking cigarettes or eating your favorite comfort foods. That stressors—large and small—affect our health is a truism. Laments like "I'm worried sick" convey the conventional wisdom that being "stressed out" will harm our health. Literally thousands of academic studies reveal that stressful life events (such as a job loss), ongoing strains (such as burdensome caregiving duties), and even daily "hassles" (such as persistent traffic jams on the commute to work) affect nearly all aspects of our physical and emotional well-being.

Yet we have all experienced stressful times—maybe a major work deadline, or relocating cross-country for a new job—when we came out unscathed, feeling not only emotionally and physically healthy, but better than we did prior to the crisis. This experience is not unique; dozens of academic studies also provide support for the rallying cry "that which doesn't kill us makes us stronger," which suggests that we may grow more resilient and resourceful with every challenge. But how can stress be a source of both compromised health and resilience? And why do some people withstand tremendous adversity without a scratch, while others fall ill or become emotionally despondent when faced with even a seemingly minor hassle?

Worried Sick answers these and other questions about how stress makes us sick and depressed and even shortens our life spans. I will also show how and why some people are resilient and seemingly immune to such health woes—even in the face of unimaginable stress. Figuring out our own sources of strength and vulnerability is an important step toward developing personal strategies to minimize stress and its unhealthy consequences. Yet I will also challenge the notion that merely reducing stress in our lives—doing deep-breathing exercises or venting to our best friend—will help us to stay healthy despite our increasingly hectic lives as workers, parents, students, and caregivers. By focusing on repairing the stressors in our lives and trying to find quick-fix solutions (a good babysitter, a new job, an antidepressant), we're missing the larger picture. Many of the stressors that we face in everyday life are not our problems alone; rather, they are symptoms of much larger, sweeping problems in contemporary U.S. society.

For instance, what might have benefited Rob most? A visit with a therapist? A prescription for an antidepressant? An economy that provided full-time jobs with benefits to all qualified workers? A culture that encouraged men to talk about their fears and insecurities, rather than keeping their feelings bottled up? And while Marisol's college advisor told her to get more sleep and attend stress-reduction workshops at her university health center, might a better solution have been programs to help first-generation college students to fund their education? Although the self-help guides lining the shelves of bookstores give us tips on how to manage our stress, and prescription medications to "cure" our anxiety are just a doctor's visit away, more sweeping solutions may be necessary.

Overview of Chapters

The following chapters delve into the concept of stress: defining what it is; explaining how it affects our emotional and physical health; identifying the biological, psychological, and economic factors that protect against (or exacerbate) the consequences of stress; and showing what can be done to minimize its impact on our everyday lives. In this first chapter, I provide a brief overview of the history and concept of "stress," and describe the diverse forms that stress may take. Although we often use the term "stress" as a catch-all to describe the many nerve-jangling experiences in life, we will see that stress can take many forms: stressful events, such as a house fire or job loss; chronic stressors that persist over time, such as marital conflict or a long-term illness; daily hassles, such as traffic jams or a misbehaving pet; and network events, or those stressors bedeviling others that may affect us, such as a spouse's work troubles or a child's difficulties at school. I also show how stress exposure varies based our personal characteristics, including gender, race, age, and social class.

In chapter 2, "Sweating the Small (and Big) Stuff: How and Why Stress Affects Our Mental Health," I describe how our mental health is affected by the stress in our lives. Feeling sad, anxious, lonely, depressed, or suicidal is rarely something that is just "in our heads." Symptoms of sadness and depression often can be traced back to a chronic or acute stressor, whether profound, such as the death of a loved one, or fleeting, such as being rejected by one's first-choice college. Yet the extent to which a stressor affects our mental health varies based on important characteristics of the stressor, such as whether it was expected or unanticipated; whether our peers are also experiencing a similar stressor; and the events that precede, co-occur with, or follow the main stressor. I summarize classic and contemporary theories on stress and mental health, and provide evidence from scientific studies showing precisely how and why stressors of modern life can overwhelm our ability to cope.

Chapter 3, "Under Our Skin: How and Why Stress Affects Our Physical Health," shows how stress affects our physical health, including our susceptibility to colds, how quickly our wounds heal, and how long we live. Early research on stress, conducted by endocrinologist Hans Selye (1956), viewed physical distress as an automatic response to any environmental stressor. In the six decades since the publication of Selye's path-breaking work, scientists working in fields ranging from genetics to psychophysiology to neuroscience have identified multiple biological pathways linking stress to physical health conditions. Social and behavioral scientists have contributed by identifying the coping tactics and health behaviors that link stress to health, such as smoking or overeating. Social scientists also have explored the ways that structural and economic factors related to stress (such as job loss and thus loss of health benefits) can indirectly affect one's health. Taken together, this research sheds light on why some health conditions, especially heart disease, are particularly susceptible to stress.

One of the most important things to know about stress is that two people may respond very differently to the exact same stressor; one person may become depressed or suicidal, while another may just accept it and move on. What accounts for these vast differences? In chapter 4, "Why Some Crumble and Others Bounce Back: Risk and Resilience in the Face of Stress," I show how some people bounce back from—and even thrive—in the face of stress and challenge, whereas others may become debilitated. In the past two decades, stress researchers have paid particular attention to "gene-environment interactions," or the ways that our genetic makeup renders us particularly resilient (or vulnerable) when faced with stress. I describe the biological, psychological, interpersonal, and socioeconomic factors that help some people to bounce back from stress, while others break under the pressure. I draw primarily on "stress process" theories developed by sociologists, which focus on resources such as personality, coping style, and interpersonal relations that shape how we respond to stress.

Literally thousands of scholarly studies show how stress hurts, so what can we do about it? In chapter 5, "Paths to Healing: Strategies for Overcoming Life's Stressors," I review strategies to minimize the health-depleting consequences of stress, and highlight which ones work and which ones don't. It is impossible to turn on the television or pick up a magazine today without seeing at least some tips to "battle stress." The past decade has seen an explosion of popular books, magazine articles, and television programs focused on reducing stress, but which ones work? And how do they work? I review the results from rigorous scientific studies and highlight those interventions, pharmaceutical treatments, or programs that have been identified as effective for battling stress-related health woes. I also show that we often cannot battle stress on our own; I highlight sweeping social factors that contribute to the stress levels of many Americans, and suggest policies to help minimize both exposure to stress and its health-depleting consequences.

WHAT IS STRESS?

A Brief History

Before we focus on the specific ways that stress affects health, it is important to first understand the basic history of and core concepts in stress research. Stress or a stressor refers to any environmental, social, biological, or psychological demand that requires a person to adjust his or her usual patterns of behavior. The notion that stress makes us sick, anxious, or depressed traces back to the 1956 classic book *The Stress of Life*, in which endocrinologist Hans Selye wrote that any harmful environmental stimulus would trigger adverse biological reactions. Selye borrowed the term "stress" from scientists in the field of engineering, who described stress as the forces that can put strain on a physical structure. For example, a scientist could exert physical force on a piece of metal in such a way that the metal could bend or even shatter like glass when it met its stress threshold. The notion that objects (and people!) can either bend or break when their stress levels reach a certain point has since been a recurring theme in research. In his early studies, Selye exposed lab animals, typically mice, to a physically distressing condition such as extreme cold or physical pain and then documented the organism's physical response. A guiding assumption of his work was that the consequences of stress were "nonspecific"; that is, regardless of what the specific stressor was (e.g., extreme cold versus starvation), it would have similar effects on the lab animal's physical response.

Although Selye was an endocrinologist who studied animals, his ideas and research set the foundation for the first wave of social science research on human responses to stress. One of the earliest social studies of stress was conducted in the 1960s by psychiatrists Thomas H. Holmes and Richard H. Rahe. They developed one of the first instruments to measure social stressors, or the types of interpersonal stressors that humans experience in everyday life. This instrument, the Social Readjustment Rating Scale (SRRS), was a questionnaire that asked people to indicate which of several dozen stressful life events they had experienced in the past twelve months. As figure 1.1 shows, life events are ranked on a scale from 0 to 100 "life change units (LCU)," meaning that some events are more serious than others, and thus may put one at more severe risk for illness or disease. An individual's self-report of stress in the past year could then be examined in relation to one's physical health symptoms, as a way to understand the association between stress and health. After subjects checked off all of the events that they had experienced in the past year, and summed up the total number of LCUs associated with those events, they could then estimate their risk of illness. For example, those with total scores of 300 or more would have an 80 percent risk of falling ill, whereas those with scores lower than 150 would have just a 30 percent risk of illness.

Just as Selye argued that the consequences of stress were "nonspecific," Holmes and Rahe also presumed that *any* change in one's social environment could overwhelm one's ability to cope, and increase vulnerability to ill health. For example, figure 1.1 shows that the "death of a spouse" rated 100 LCUs on the SRSS, whereas an "outstanding personal achievement" rated 28 LCUs. However, the SRSS did not consider that the former is almost always interpreted by the bereaved spouse to be a sad, devastating, and life-altering event, whereas the latter is typically interpreted as a pleasant and desired experience. Rather, the assumption stood that each life change would have a health-depleting effect, and that the events merely differed with respect to the magnitude of their effects. As Holmes and Rahe wrote, "change in one's life requires an effort to adapt and then to regain stability. This process probably saps energy the body would ordinarily use to maintain itself, so susceptibility to illness increases." In other words, all changes were viewed as potentially harmful, regardless of one's interpretation of change (e.g., was it desired or not?), how long the stressful period lasted, and a range of other conditions that could make the transition more or less distressing.

Contemporary Concepts and Measures

Contemporary research on stress has abandoned the assumption that "all change is harmful," and instead recognizes tremendous variation in how we might experience, interpret, and respond to stress. First, researchers have moved away from using the general term "stress" and instead consider the specific forms that stress takes. The main subtypes identified are life events, chronic strains, daily hassles, and network events.

Life events are acute changes that require adjustment within a relatively short time period, such as being laid off from one's job, the death of a spouse, or losing one's home in a fire. Life events often signify a transition between two statuses or roles, such as the movement from spouse to widow, worker to ex-worker, or able-bodied person to disabled. One particular subtype, traumatic life events, such as experiencing a sexual assault, have especially harmful and long-lasting effects on health. In general, the health impact of a stressful life event depends on its magnitude (i.e., how serious is it?), desirability (i.e., was the change desired or not?), expectedness (i.e., was it anticipated or was it a surprise?), and timing (i.e., how old were you when it occurred?). In general, events that are unexpected are particularly distressing. For example, if one loses their job suddenly and without warning, it may be a jarring "shock to the system," and one may be ill-prepared to find a new job. However, if one sees his or her colleagues being laid off, that worker might start looking for a new position to help prepare for the inevitability of one's own job loss.

Life events that happen "off-time," meaning earlier or later than is typical, also are considered particularly harmful. For example, having a baby may be a source of great joy, yet the changes that new parenthood impose may have harmful consequences for one's emotional and physical health. Sleep deprivation, worries about caring for a baby, changes in one's daily routines, and a renegotiation of one's marital roles can take a personal toll. Yet for someone who undergoes the parenthood transition earlier than expected, such as the teen moms featured on "reality" shows like MTV's *16 and Pregnant* or *Teen Mom*, the transition may be particularly stressful. The young mother typically is not prepared for her role, may not have a group of peers who can support her, and may even face stigmatization and the loss of social support of friends and teachers who feel that teenagers should not become parents. As a result, the transition to parenthood may be more stressful for those who experience the life event "off-time."

The health effects of stressful events involving a transition out of a social role, such as loss of a job or a marriage, are contingent on one's role history or on the qualitative aspects of the role

FIGURE 1.1.

Holmes-Rahe Social Readjustment Scale (1967)

Place a tick next to each event that has occurred to you
in the last 12 months.

Event	Yes or No	Scale of Impact
Death of a spouse		100
Divorce		73
Marital separation		65
Jail term		63
Death of a close family member		63
Personal injury or illness		53
Marriage		50
Fired at work		47
Marital reconciliation		45
Retirement		45
Change in health of family member		44
Pregnancy		40
Sex difficulties		39
Gain of a new family member		39
Business readjustment		39
Change in financial state		38
Death of a close friend		37
Change to a different line of work		36
Change in number of arguments with spouse		35
Mortgage over $150,000		31
Foreclosure of mortgage or loan		30
Change in responsibilities at work		29
Son or daughter leaving home		29
Trouble with in-laws		29

FIGURE I.I.

Holmes-Rahe Social Readjustment Scale (1967) (continued)

Event	Yes or No	Scale of Impact
Outstanding personal achievement		28
Partner begins or stops work		26
Begin or end school		26
Change in living conditions		25
Revision of personal habits		24
Trouble with boss		23
Change in work hours or conditions		20
Change in residence		20
Change in schools		20
Change in recreation		19
Change in church activities		19
Change in social activities		18
Mortgage or loan less than $150,000		17
Change in sleeping habits		16
Change in number of family get-togethers		15
Change in eating habits		15
Vacation		13
Christmas		12
Minor violations of the law		11

Total up your points. If you scored over 300 you may have increased risk of developing health difficulties as a result of coping with multiple stressful events in your life.

SOURCE: Holmes, T. A., & Rahe, R.H. (1967). The social readjustment rating scale. *Journal of Psychosomatic Research,* 11, 213–18.

one is exiting or entering. Divorce from an abusive spouse or being fired from an intolerable job may actually enhance one's happiness and self-esteem. By the same token, the loss of a particularly cherished role, such as forced retirement from a job one loved, may be especially distressing.

Scholars have recently proposed that individuals might also experience distress because of an event or role transition that they anticipated but that never came to fruition. The concept of a "nonevent" is fairly new but is one that most of us can relate to. Imagine being passed over for a much-desired promotion at work. Or think about forty-five-year-old Dawn. Although she always dreamed of finding the perfect husband, buying a home with a white picket fence, and having an adorable child or two, Dawn is now single, childless, and has few romantic prospects in the rural town where she works as a schoolteacher. She struggles daily with sadness, loneliness, and worries of "growing old alone." Researchers are only starting to investigate the ways that *not* experiencing an event that one had desired can take a toll on health and well-being. Preliminary evidence suggests that not experiencing a family transition—such as a marriage or first birth—within a few years of the "typical" age for doing so can heighten one's feelings of depression.

Whereas life events are generally thought of as single point-in-time transitions, chronic strains are persistent and repeated demands that require us to adapt, often over long periods of time. Think about being trapped in an unhappy marriage, having a stressful job, or living in a dangerous crime-ridden neighborhood; each of these conditions stays with us, day after day. That's partly why chronic strains are considered more harmful than life events; they are constant and often reflect situations that we cannot easily change or escape.

Researchers tend to classify chronic strains into three types: status, role, and ambient strains. Status strains arise out of one's position in the social hierarchies that are present in all societies.

For example, in the United States, a history of racial stratification and discrimination has created a hierarchy in which African Americans tend to have less political and economic power than whites. Similarly, for much of U.S. history, women have held less power and had fewer resources than men. Belonging to a socially or economically disadvantaged group may create daily challenges that threaten our health.

Role strains are conflicts or demands related to social roles, such as juggling work and family responsibilities. Sociologists often write about role overload, or the ways that our multiple responsibilities may pile up and threaten our physical or emotional well-being. As Naomi's experiences revealed earlier in this chapter, simultaneously caring for her terminally ill husband, her elderly mother, and her young-adult children subjected Naomi to physical wear and tear. Within a year of the deaths of her husband and mother, Naomi had a stroke. Role strains may also threaten one's emotional well-being. The Internet is home to countless "mommy bloggers" who write daily about the guilt and anxiety they feel as they juggle jobs, childrearing, and marriage—with many feeling that they're floundering on all fronts. National surveys by the Gallup Organization also show that roughly half of all Americans feel that they don't have time to do all they need to do each day, and they feel stressed as a result. As we might expect, working parents are most likely to report the pressures of time.

Ambient strains refer to stressful aspects of the physical environment, such as noise or pollution. Environmental scientists have long known that exposure to pollution, traffic, or worries about neighborhood crime can erode one's defenses and make one vulnerable to sickness. Yet in recent years, scientists have discovered that other aspects of the physical environment, including noise, can chip away at one's health and wellness. Noise is more than just an annoyance; recent studies show that persons living in loud neighborhoods with noisy traffic have more sleep troubles, and consequently their health suffers. In fact, one recent study found that every additional ten decibels of noise from traffic is linked with a 12 percent increased risk of a heart attack.

Even those fortunate enough to enjoy rewarding jobs, safe neighborhoods, and happy marriages aren't completely immune to stress exposure. Contemporary studies conclude that even minor nuisances, if experienced repeatedly for long periods of time, can threaten our health and happiness. Daily hassles such as traffic tie-ups, a neighbor's barking dog, or subway delays on one's commute to work are minor and seemingly insignificant occurrences that require adjustment throughout the day. Historically, most stress research focused on "major" stressors such as life events and chronic strains, although in recent years researchers have begun to collect daily diary reports of hassles throughout the day, and find clear linkages between these "quotidian" strains and well-being. Not surprisingly, these effects are much more modest than the effects of chronic strains or traumatic events; the former tend to dissipate in a day or two.

Although the three types of stressors (events, chronic strains, and hassles) often are described as distinctive and discrete experiences, a stressor rarely occurs in isolation. Eminent sociologist and stress researcher Leonard Pearlin describes this process as stress proliferation, in which "people exposed to a serious adversity [are] at risk for later exposure to additional adversities." For example, a divorce may trigger a chain of new and chronic strains, such as financial worries, complex child custody arrangements, and balancing single parenthood with work and dating. Conversely, chronic strains may precede and even give rise to a stressful life event. For example, marriage to a husband who is abusive or has substance use problems is inherently stressful, and also may lead the wife to initiate a divorce, thus creating a new cycle of stressors.

Stress from one life domain also may "spill over" to create stress in another domain. For example, difficulties at work, such as an unrealistically demanding boss or relentless deadlines, may "spill over" to our family lives, limiting the time and attention we can give to loved ones. Similarly, stressful experiences in one person's life may spill over or "cross over" to affect others in the social network. A network event, such as an adult child's imprisonment or a brother's persistent unemployment, may affect our own mental health, whether through the distress of witnessing a loved one suffer, or because we must take on added responsibilities to help them through their difficult time (e.g., serving as a custodial grandparent if one's child is imprisoned). Our network members' stressful encounters may also challenge our identities in potentially distressing ways. Take sixty-eight-year-old Beverly, for example. Beverly was a stay-at-home mother for many years, and prided herself on having provided a safe and loving home for her four children. As her children became adults, each encountered serious problems, including drug abuse, a bitter divorce and custody battle, and unemployment. Studies show that parents like Beverly may feel personally responsible for their children's problems, and their confidence, self-worth, and emotional well-being may suffer as a result.

A final way that others' experiences may affect our own health is through a phenomenon called "stress contagion." This is a process whereby one person's reaction to stress affects the health of a significant other, such as when one spouse's depression following a job loss compromises the other spouse's well-being. Just as a common cold and chicken pox are contagious and can spread from person to person, emotional distress also can spread through social networks. Although the exact processes are unclear, sociologist and physician Nicholas Christakis and his colleagues have started to document the ways that distress can "travel" through social networks. For example, Christakis and his colleagues found that depressive symptoms in one person could "spread" to neighbors, siblings, and friends. One explanation for this emotional contagion is that our lives are often similar to those of our significant others, and thus we experience the same sources of stress and joy. Yet another plausible explanation is, simply put, that it's depressing to see our favorite people depressed.

WHO EXPERIENCES STRESS?

Everyone experiences stress, but some people experience more intense, frequent, harmful, and uncontrollable stressors than others. We've all heard an acquaintance bemoan how "stressed" they are because they have two party invitations for the same evening, or that their teenage child is "stressed out" about whether to accept an offer of admission from Harvard or from Haverford. These stressors are often snidely referred to as "good problems to have" or "first-world problems." By contrast, we might also have an acquaintance like Louie, who earned minimum wage as a house painter, suffered an injury at work, and consequently lost his job because he could no longer climb ladders and paint homes. With limited savings and meager disability pay, someone like Louie might have foreclosed on his home, or worse yet, found himself unable to pay rent for even a run-down apartment. It would be hard for even the most optimistic Pollyanna to describe such stressors as "good problems to have."

These vignettes illustrate an important theme of stress research: exposure to stress is not randomly distributed throughout the population, but is highly structured and reflects patterns of inequality. The types of stress we experience vary by our social locations, including our social class, age, race, ethnicity, and gender. As we will see in subsequent chapters, each of these factors affects not only our exposure to stress but also the resources that help us to cope.

The social stratification of stress is a complex process. In this section, I'll briefly point out a few ways that the types of stressors to which we're exposed vary based on our personal characteristics. Overall, when Americans are asked to name the leading sources of stress in their life, the majority name financial worries, work, money, personal relationships, and family responsibilities. Each year, the American Psychological Association (APA) carries out a survey of more than one thousand Americans and finds that although there are slight changes from year to year in our leading sources of stress, financial issues, work, and family consistently rank at the top of the list (see figure 1.2).

However, when researchers break down the U.S. population into subgroups, they start to see some variation in the stressors that plague us. Women, for example, historically have suffered the "costs of caring" and experience more stress related to marriage, childrearing, work-family overload, and network events. Men, on average, have been more vulnerable to financial and job-related stressors. These patterns reflect the ways that gender has guided the allocation of social roles through much of the twentieth century, with women historically "specializing" in childrearing and men taking on the role of primary breadwinner. However, these differences may converge as women increasingly become the family's main breadwinner, and men increasingly take on roles of primary parent and caretaker. Racial and ethnic minorities are more likely than whites to experience stressors related to their minority status, including discrimination and interpersonal mistreatment on the grounds of their ethnic background. Given a history of racial stratification in the United States, blacks and Latinos are particularly susceptible to stressors such as economic strains, long-term unemployment, poverty, physically dangerous work conditions, and the anxieties associated with living in unsafe neighborhoods.

The types of stressors we experience also shift as we age. Older adults tend to experience stress related to their own and their spouse's declining health, caregiving strains, the deaths of spouses and peers, and difficulties negotiating their physical environment, especially for those with physical limitations. Working-age adults typically rate financial troubles, work stress, parenting concerns, and marital difficulties as their main sources of stress, whereas for children and teens, stress is often generated by the words and deeds of others. School bullies, critical school teachers, unhappily married parents, and difficult siblings often are a source of distress for school-age youth.

Despite the importance of gender, race, and age to stress exposure, most researchers agree that the single most powerful determinant of both one's exposure and one's responses to stress is

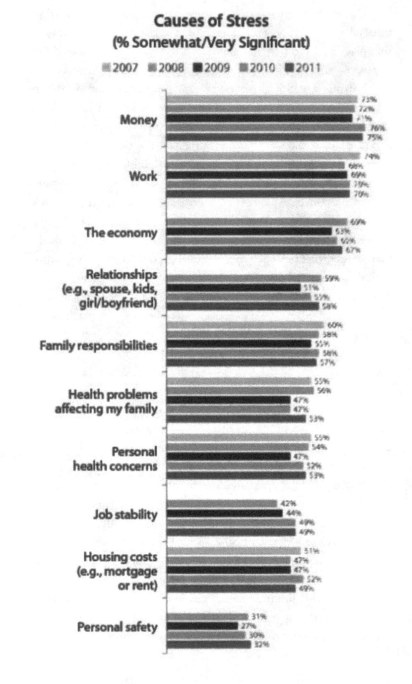

Causes of Stress
(% Somewhat/Very Significant)

2007   2008   2009   2010   2011

Money: 73%, 72%, 71%, 76%, 75%

Work: 74%, 68%, 69%, 70%, 70%

The economy: 69%, 63%, 66%, 67%

Relationships (e.g., spouse, kids, girl/boyfriend): 59%, 51%, 55%, 58%

Family responsibilities: 60%, 58%, 55%, 58%, 57%

Health problems affecting my family: 55%, 56%, 47%, 47%, 53%

Personal health concerns: 55%, 54%, 47%, 52%, 53%

Job stability: 42%, 44%, 49%, 49%

Housing costs (e.g., mortgage or rent): 51%, 47%, 47%, 52%, 49%

Personal safety: 31%, 27%, 30%, 32%

social class or socioeconomic status (SES). Socioeconomic status refers to one's place in the social hierarchy, where the tiers are defined by one's economic and social power. Socioeconomic status encompasses one's level of education, the status or prestige of one's occupation, how much money one has to live on (income), and the value of one's possessions (assets). Low SES increases one's risk of stressful life events, ranging from divorce to job loss to early onset of health problems, as well as chronic stressors, including overcrowded or dilapidated living conditions, marital strife, and discrimination. As we will see in chapter 3, SES also is negatively related to important resources that we need to manage stress, including supportive social ties, access to health care, and financial reserves that can provide a buffer during times of strain.

The high levels of stress experienced by those with limited socioeconomic resources partially explains why poorer people in the United States have a higher risk of just about every major illness and a higher risk of premature death than those with richer economic resources. As stressors accumulate, our ability to adapt can be overwhelmed, depleting our psychological and physical reserves, and increasing the chances of illness, injury, or depression. Although Holmes and Rahe's SRSS scale has fallen out of favor with contemporary stress researchers because of its simplistic approach to conceptualizing stress, most experts recognize that Holmes and Rahe did get one thing right: the accumulation of multiple severe stressors can overwhelm our minds and bodies, and increase our risk of mental and physical health problems. In the next three chapters, I show exactly how these effects unfold, for whom, and the resources that may help to mitigate their harmful consequences.

Figure 1.2.
Top Sources of Stress in the United States, 2011 (Source: APA, 2012).
Base: All respondents 2007 (n=1848); 2008 (n=1791); ; 2009 (n=1568); 2010 (n=1134); 2011 (n=1226). Q625: Below is a list of things people say cause stress in their lives. For each one, please indicate how significant a source of stress it is in your life.

CHAPTER 2

Sweating the Small
(and Big) Stuff

How and Why Stress Affects
Our Mental Health

EVERYONE HAS HAD AN occasional "bad day" when they wake up feeling blue, cranky, or fearful of what the day holds in store. Often, these feelings fade quickly and are chalked up to "waking up on the wrong side of the bed." Yet for people undergoing high levels of stress in their daily lives, feeling sad, anxious, angry, or depressed is rarely something that is just "in our heads." Intense and persistent symptoms of depression, anxiety, and even anger often can be traced back to stress, whether events are life-altering, such as the death of a loved one, or fleeting, such as a looming deadline on a major work assignment. For those experiencing overwhelming stress, such as military combat or sexual assault, the psychological consequences can be even more severe.

Why and how does stress affect our mental health? Which aspects of mental health are affected most profoundly? Are some stressors particularly damaging? How long do these effects last? Why might some people react to stress by feeling depressed, while others become angry or anxious? In this chapter I summarize classic and contemporary theories on stress and mental health, and describe both the psychosocial and biological explanations of how stress can harm us. I provide evidence from recent studies showing precisely how stress may rob us of our emotional well being, as well as a handful of studies that document psychological growth in the face of personal challenges. Before delving into the questions of why and how stress affects mental health, I provide a brief review of precisely what mental health is, how stress researchers document linkages between stress and mental health, which symptoms may be particularly susceptible to the stressors in our lives, and the reasons why different people react with different symptoms.

What Is Mental Health and How Do We Study It?

Mental health refers to one's emotional well-being and absence of mental health disorders. However, stress researchers are more likely to discuss mental health problems rather than emotional wellness. Part of the reason for this emphasis on mental health problems is that stress researchers are interested in identifying and ultimately eradicating the negative psychological consequences of stress. Stress researchers also tend to focus on mental health symptoms that could afflict almost any person at a particularly difficult time in their lives; these symptoms generally include depression, anxiety, anger, and grief. A growing number of scholars also explore more intense outcomes, such as suicidality or post-traumatic stress disorder, which may afflict persons exposed to extreme stress. (Stress researchers also examine harmful strategies individuals adopt to soothe their emotional distress, including drinking and overeating; I discuss these and other health behaviors in chapter 3.)

Stress researchers typically do not focus on major mental illnesses that may have a strong genetic component. Such disorders, including bipolar disorder (i.e., manic depression) or schizophrenia may be triggered by a major stressor or by living in a stressful environment, but stress alone (in absence of family history of mental illness) is typically not sufficient to "cause" schizophrenia or manic depression. Additionally, many stress researchers conduct their studies by using large surveys of the U.S. population, measuring exposure to stress, and documenting statistical associations between one's stressful experiences and responses to checklists that capture one's symptoms of depression, anger, or anxiety (for an example, see figure 2.1). Because major mental health disorders such as bipolar disorder and schizophrenia affect relatively small populations (4 and <1 percent of the U.S. population, respectively), most researchers would not find a sufficient number of cases to examine in a survey study. Persons with major mental health conditions also are unlikely to complete the survey they've been given. (A full discussion of complex conditions such as schizophrenia is beyond the scope of this book, although the National Institute of Mental Health has helpful resources for understanding these conditions. See nimh.nih.gov.)

Mental health symptoms may be general responses to stress, meaning that they may be triggered by a broad range of possible events and experiences, or specific, meaning that they may be triggered by a much narrower set of stressors. Three of the most common general symptoms or conditions studied by stress researchers are depression, anxiety, and anger. Think about the times you've sighed and said, "I'm so depressed," or clenched your fists and growled, "I'm so mad I could scream." On other occasions, you might have lamented, "I'm on pins and needles," or, even worse, "I'm a nervous wreck." Think about the major events in your life at that time, or even trivial hassles on the days when you've uttered these words; you can probably recall dozens of different events or experiences that contributed to your feelings of depression, anger, or anxiety. Scientific research concurs that a broad range of acute and chronic stressors contribute to

FIGURE 2.1.

Center for Epidemiologic Studies Depression Scale (Radloff, 1977)

Below is a list of some of the ways you may have felt or behaved. Please indicate how often you've felt this way during the past week.

Place a check mark in the appropriate column. During the past week . . .	Rarely or none of the time (less than 1 day)	Some or a little of the time (1–2 days)	Occasionally or a moderate amount of time (3–4 days)	All of the time (5 7 days)
1. I was bothered by things that usually don't bother me.				
2. I did not feel like eating; my appetite was poor.				
3. I felt that I could not shake off the blues even with help from my family.				
4. I felt that I was just as good as other people.				
5. I had trouble keeping my mind on what I was doing.				
6. I felt depressed.				
7. I felt that everything I did was an effort.				
8. I felt hopeful about the future.				
9. I thought my life had been a failure.				
10. I felt fearful.				
11. My sleep was restless.				
12. I was happy.				
13. I talked less than usual.				
14. I felt lonely.				
15. People were unfriendly.				
16. I enjoyed life.				
17. I had crying spells.				
18. I felt sad.				
19. I felt that people disliked me.				
20. I could not 'get going.'				

NOTE: Items 4, 8, 12, and 16 are reverse-coded when calculating one's final depressive symptoms score.

SOURCE: Radloff, L.S. (1977). The CES-D scale: A self-report depression scale for research in the general population. *Applied Psychological Measurement, 1:* 385–401.

those general symptoms. By contrast, some symptoms are very specific to a particular stressful context; the most widely studied one is grief, which is a direct emotional response to the loss of a person or object to which we were deeply attached emotionally. Symptoms of grief tend to be triggered by very specific losses, such as the death of a family member.

General Symptoms

DEPRESSION. Phrases like "I'm so depressed" or "That movie was *so* depressing" are a part of our daily vocabularies, yet many of us do not know precisely what depression entails. Many believe that "depressed" simply means "sad," yet that would be an incomplete characterization. Depression has four components: emotional, cognitive, motivational, and somatic symptoms. The emotional aspects of depression include the sad mood and diminished pleasure that almost always accompany depression. Cognitive components include the ways that our thought processes change when we are depressed; we may develop a very bleak view of the world and may become hopeless about the future or may believe that we are worthless. The motivational component of depression is linked to our behaviors; it is often difficult to get motivated or to take action when one is depressed. Depressed people often struggle with getting out of bed in the morning. Finally, somatic aspects of depression are physical conditions, such as fatigue, headaches, or sleeping too much or too little.

Different people may experience different symptoms; for instance, women are more likely to report emotional symptoms like feeling sad or crying, whereas men may not report such feelings and instead say that they view the future as hopeless. Researchers have argued that the types of symptoms that people report on depression symptom checklists are consistent with socialization processes; men who were raised to hide their feelings may not admit that they feel sad or that they have cried, yet may be more likely to report other aspects of depression. This distinction is important for both clinicians and laypersons to recognize; depression in men often goes undetected (and untreated) because they do not easily admit to others that they are feeling sad and blue.

Depression is the most widely studied mental health outcome in stress research. There are at least three reasons why so many of the studies that you will read about in this book focus on depression. First, depression is one of the most common mental health diagnoses in psychiatry, and one of the most common mental health problems documented in the U.S. population. Recent studies estimate that about 16 percent of Americans have ever suffered from a major depressive disorder (MDD), and about 7 percent have experienced MDD in the past year. Major depressive disorder (MDD) occurs when a person has experienced severe depressive symptoms for a period of two weeks or more. These severe symptoms interfere with a person's ability to work, sleep, study, eat, and enjoy once-pleasurable activities. However, a much larger proportion of Americans may experience at least a few symptoms for a period of two weeks or more, a condition referred to as subclinical depression or minor depression. Although the latter is less serious than MDD, it is still a source of concern. Depressive symptoms may affect people's ability to go to work, to maintain high-quality relationships, and to be effective parents. Policy makers have noted that depression accounts for more workplace absenteeism and more costly losses in worker productivity than any other illness. Persons who suffer from even minor depressive symptoms may be at risk for MDD if they encounter additional stressors in their lives.

Second, depression is a common outcome in stress research because it is a response to many stressful experiences that social scientists find most pressing. Scholars dating back to Sigmund Freud have observed that depression is a reaction to loss or "exit events." It may arise in response to the loss of an important social role (e.g., retirement), a significant other (e.g., widowhood), one's home and community (e.g., displacement following a fire), or even the loss of feelings of competence (e.g., having a business venture fail). Depression and hopelessness also may result when one feels overwhelmed, trapped, or fearful about the accumulation of stress in one's life. In other words, depressive symptoms may emerge in the face of the broad range of stressful events, chronic stressors, network events, and daily strains.

Finally, depressive symptoms are relatively easy to measure in the general population, so scientists can relate individuals' reports of stress with their reports of depressive symptoms. One of the most commonly used instruments for measuring depressive symptoms in population-based studies is the Center for Epidemiologic Studies Depression Scale (CES-D) designed in the 1970s by Lenore Radloff. This twenty-item checklist is shown in figure 2.1; the symptoms included in this measure reflect the four subcomponents discussed earlier: emotional, somatic, motivational, and cognitive. Researchers calculate a score for each individual, based on how many symptoms they report, and how frequently they experience each symptom. Persons scoring in the highest range are considered at risk for major depression. Other instruments are widely used to assess MDD in the population, including the Composite *International Diagnostic Interview (CIDI)* and the Diagnostic Interview Schedule (DIS). While the CESD shows one's level of symptoms on a scale from none to many, tools such as the CIDI and MDD classify persons based on whether or not they have clinically significant depression.

This research approach helps scholars to document the depressive consequences of stress in the overall U.S. population. For example, a 2013 Gallup-Healthways survey of more than 100,000 Americans found that 10 percent have a current diagnosis of depression, yet this rate is as high as 17 percent among those who are unemployed. Many scholars believe that this population-based approach provides the most accurate portrait of the consequences of stress. Research approaches that examine stress and mental health in clinical populations, or in those populations already seeking psychiatric care, may overstate the harmful emotional effects of stress precisely because their studies are focused on those who by definition are suffering from a mental health problem.

A vivid example of this is Judith Wallerstein's classic study *The Unexpected Legacy of Divorce*. Wallerstein, a clinical psychologist, concluded that children whose parents divorced when they were young were more depressed and anxious, and that these mental health woes followed them into adulthood, compromising their own romantic relationships. However, Wallerstein's findings partly reflect the fact that she studied children who were already receiving psychological care to help them with the stress of their parents' divorce. By contrast, studies based on population-based samples find that most children of divorce do just fine after the early months of the stressful transition have passed.

ANXIETY. Anxiety includes unsettling feelings and emotions, as well as physical responses and behaviors associated with nervousness. Feelings might include worry, tension, and dread, whereas physical symptoms might include muscle tension, heart palpitations, difficulty breathing, heightened blood pressure, and sweating. Behavioral symptoms might include being easily excitable and "jumpy." Extreme forms of anxiety might include panic attacks or even phobias (i.e., extreme and illogical fears). Anxiety disorders are very common in the United States today, with more than 18 percent of the U.S. population having such a condition in the past year, and fully 30 percent ever experiencing an anxiety disorder in their lifetime. Most of the research discussed in this book focuses on more modest symptoms, such as nervousness, rather than full-blown anxiety or panic disorders.

Researchers have debated whether anxiety is triggered by the same types of stressors as depression. This debate is difficult to resolve, because many people who experience depression also experience anxiety; this co-occurrence of symptoms is referred to as "comorbidity." Stressful events and experiences that generate fear and anxiety may also be associated with experiences that trigger depression. For instance, upon the death of a spouse, a widow or widower may feel deep sadness over the loss of a beloved partner, yet may also feel anxious about the new challenges that lie ahead as a single person—such as living alone or managing all the household tasks that were previously performed by the spouse.

Psychologists have documented that mild symptoms of anxiety might serve a positive function. Moderate levels of anxiety keep people on their toes, enabling them to juggle multiple tasks and putting them on high alert for potential problems. Just think about the last time you had to give a public talk or had a big exam; a bit of nerves on the days leading up to the event might have pushed you to prepare for the big day. However, extreme symptoms of anxiety are problematic because they make even simple tasks much more difficult. This notion that low levels of anxiety can be beneficial dates back to the early twentieth century, when Harvard psychologists Robert Yerkes and John Dodson hypothesized that "arousal" (or a slight elevation of stress hormones) enhances performance—but only to a point. When anxiety gets too high, performance suffers instead. Contemporary work finds support for what is called the Yerkes-Dodson curve; this is an upside-down U-shaped curve showing a curvilinear association between anxiety and performance on tasks such as learning. However, as we know from our own experiences, when our nerves get the better of us, we become flustered and make mistakes—often making ourselves even more anxious. In this way, living in a constant state of stress-induced anxiety may lead to a spiraling out of secondary stressors as we struggle to maintain order and a sense of competence in our lives.

ANGER Anger is an important emotional consequence of stress, although relatively little research focuses on these symptoms. Anger generally encompasses disturbing feelings such as frustration, annoyance, hostility, and even rage. While depression is often a response to stressors involving loss, and anxiety is related to stressors where uncertainty is high, anger is associated with experiences deemed unfair or unjust. For instance, experiences of discrimination in the workplace, such as being fired unfairly, or losing a child to murder, are likely to elicit anger more than sadness. Anger is a particularly harmful reaction to stress, because those who are angry may build a wall between themselves and the very people who can offer them support and assistance. Whereas depression and anxiety symptoms may signal to friends and family that one is in distress and in need of help, the hostility that accompanies anger often pushes away those important sources of support. As we will see in chapter 4, social support can be an important buffer against the harmful consequences of stress.

Anger, like depression and anxiety, is often measured with symptom checklists. Men are more likely than women to show anger in the face of stress, although it is not clear whether this reflects biological factors (such as testosterone) or gender differences in how people complete anger symptom checklists. Men may be more likely to report feelings of anger and to behave in angry ways, such as aggressing against others. Women, by contrast, may be hesitant to admit feeling angry. Just as men (who are raised to be "strong and silent") may be reluctant to report crying or feeling sad when asked about their depressive symptoms, women who were raised to be docile and accommodating may not express their anger. As a result, studies may not show a strong association between stress and anger among women, yet these results may reflect only the anger expressed rather than the anger women feel privately and silently.

Specific Outcomes: Grief

The death of a loved one is considered the single most stressful event that individuals experience, as we saw in the Holmes and Rahe SRRS checklist in chapter 1. Although bereaved persons often experience feelings of depression, anxiety, and anger, they also experience the specific mental health outcome of grief. Grief is a collection of emotional symptoms that are related directly to the loss of a loved one. At the core of grief are symptoms of yearning, or longing for and wanting to reconnect with the deceased person. In addition to feelings of sadness and loss, grief also may encompass symptoms such as anxiety about the future, anger, shock, despair, and intrusive thoughts. Intrusive thoughts are symptoms similar to post-traumatic stress disorder (PTSD), in which unprovoked painful thoughts about the deceased haunt the survivor. The specific symptoms are closely tied to the nature of the death. Deaths that are deemed unfair, such as those due to medical error, are associated with symptoms of anger, whereas sudden deaths tend to trigger feelings of emotional shock. Widows and widowers who had particularly loving and close marriages tend to yearn more for the deceased than do persons who had problematic marriages.

For most bereaved persons, grief symptoms typically fade within the first six to twenty-four months after the loss, although the death of a child or a particularly traumatic death (such as a suicide or murder) is associated with much-longer-lived and intense symptoms. Roughly 5 percent of bereaved persons suffer from a severe and prolonged cluster of symptoms called "complicated grief"; these persons are incapable of resuming normal activities and responsibilities, and may be at a heightened risk for physical health problems.

Extreme Outcomes: Suicidality and
Post-Traumatic Stress Disorder

In rare cases, stress has devastating and even lethal consequences. One of the most dire outcomes of stress is suicide, or taking one's own life. Suicides are relatively rare in the United States, so stress researchers often study suicidal ideation, which refers to one's frequent thoughts about suicide or the desire to take one's own life. Although suicide rates are low in the United States, they have risen dramatically in recent years, especially among middle-aged adults belonging to the Baby Boom cohort. In 2010, the number of deaths due to suicide was roughly equal to the number of deaths due to automobile accidents (roughly 38,000 each). Men typically have much higher rates of suicide than do women.

Can stress trigger an outcome as extreme as suicide? The answer is complex. One of the most powerful precursors of suicide is MDD (major depressive disorder). Although MDD is often caused by stress, it may also be caused by biological factors related to brain chemistry. Depression, and subsequently suicide, may also be a consequence of incurable terminal illness, which may lessen one's desire to live. Suicide is also closely linked to drug and alcohol use. Persons who drink heavily, use opiates, or take intravenous drugs have suicide rates anywhere from three to eighteen times higher than those who do not abuse substances. Of course, one reason why users turn to opioid drugs like Oxy-Contin is that they are under tremendous stress and hope to soothe their pain with medication. Given how intricately tied stress, depression, substance use, and suicide are, it is difficult for researchers to definitively say that stress "causes" suicide.

However, mental health researchers and historians alike have documented one clear-cut trend: suicide rates tend to increase during times of economic recession, as they did during the Great Depression of the 1930s and the recent recession of the

2000s. As we saw in chapter 1, Rob, the forty-seven-year-old repairman, shot and killed himself after struggling emotionally with a two-year bout of unemployment. Those facing persistent unemployment, especially men whose identities are tied to the "good provider" role, may feel hopeless and suicidal after searching fruitlessly for work and struggling to support their families. Yet there are millions of Americans who lose their jobs or suffer financial devastation who do not kill themselves. Research shows that having the means to take one's life is an important factor in whether stress ultimately leads to suicide. Imagine that Rob was a gun aficionado and avid hunter; access to guns in his home would place him at a much higher risk of suicide than a peer who didn't have such means.

Another extreme outcome that has captured the interest of stress researchers in the past decade is post-traumatic stress disorder (PTSD). Those who go through extreme trauma, such as sexual assault, military combat, persistent child abuse, or even witnessing a devastating event at close hand—such as the collapse of the Twin Towers on 9/11—may experience fear and terror even when they are in safe situations. Symptoms of PTSD include reliving the traumatic events and associated physical symptoms (e.g., flashbacks and cold sweats), emotional numbness and avoidance, and being nervous and continuously "on edge." Not all people who experience severe trauma go on to experience PTSD; those at greatest risk may have a particular genetic predisposition, a history of mental health problems, or other traits that make them particularly vulnerable. Risk of PTSD is also linked to how intense the trauma was; particularly brutal or bloody bouts of combat would be more distressing to a soldier during wartime than having a desk job would be.

Not surprisingly, PTSD rates vary widely based on one's personal experiences. An estimated 4 percent of men and 10 percent of women have ever experienced PTSD, while roughly 2 and 5 percent, respectively, have had PTSD symptoms in the past year. In stark contrast, roughly one in three veterans of the Iraq and Afghanistan wars has been treated for PTSD. However, some critics of the PTSD diagnosis question whether actual rates of PTSD are increasing, or whether we live in a world today where people (and especially soldiers) are more likely than in the past to openly discuss their fears, feelings, and anxieties.

Positive Psychological Consequences of Stress

Can stress have positive consequences for our emotional health? The bulk of evidence shows that stress undermines well-being, yet emerging research on "post-traumatic growth" suggests that in some instances stress may give rise to positive outcomes, especially personal growth, as individuals recognize that they can survive and thrive in the face of difficulties. A case in point is Eric LeGrand, a twenty-year-old football player at Rutgers University who collided with an opponent when playing Army in a game in October 2010. The injury paralyzed LeGrand from the waist down, and doctors doubted that he would regain movement and functioning. While this loss would be devastating to many, LeGrand fought his way through treatment, regained some upper-body movement, and is now an author and motivational speaker who seeks to inspire others—all while confined to his wheelchair.

LeGrand's inspiring story raises the question of how and why some people can thrive in the face of life-changing adversity. A special 2004 issue of the journal *Psychological Inquiry* focused on the then-new concept of post-traumatic growth (PTG), and clarified that PTG is distinct from resilience. Resilient people may withstand a major stressor and suffer no psychological harm, or may experience mental health symptoms in the short term, but eventually return to their precrisis level of psychological health. By contrast, PTG involves suffering in the face of a crisis but ultimately enjoying psychological, interpersonal, and spiritual well-being levels that may be superior to one's precrisis levels.

Researchers have identified five positive changes associated with PTG. First, people surviving major crises may develop a sense that new opportunities have emerged from the struggle, and may envision new possibilities for their future. Second, personal relationships may be strengthened, where some feel an increased sense of connection to and empathy toward others who have suffered. Third, "survivors" may recognize their own psychological strength. For example, people who survive cancer often say things like, "If I can survive cancer, I can face anything." Fourth, those who withstand profound stress may develop a fuller appreciation of the "small" things in their lives, including personal relationships. Finally, individuals may undergo a change in their beliefs, especially their spiritual or religious views, in such a way that helps them to cope with future stressors.

Although theoretical arguments regarding post-traumatic growth are intuitively appealing, empirical evidence to date is limited. If positive effects of stress are detected, they typically are not evident until significant time has elapsed since the stressful period. For example, studies of bereavement have found that older widows who had been most dependent on their spouses during marriage had the greatest increases in self-esteem and personal growth post-loss, yet this did not emerge until nearly two years after the death.

How and Why Does Stress Affect Us?

How and why does stress make us depressed, anxious, angry, or grief-stricken? There is no silver-bullet answer. Explanations vary widely based on scientists' disciplinary training. Sociologists and epidemiologists tend to focus on the strain inherent in particular social roles, statuses, and relations. Psychologists emphasize cognitive processes and individual-level strengths and vulnerabilities. And biological scientists and neuroscientists focus on physiological pathways linking stress to mental health. No one perspective offers a complete explanation of the well–documented linkages between stress and mental health. Rather, a complex set of methodological, social, psychological, and biological factors explain these associations. In this section, I describe some of the most widely accepted explanations for why stressful events and experiences impede individuals' mental health, even if only in the short term.

Methodological Explanations

Hundreds of studies show that people who experience frequent and intense stressors experience more mental health symptoms than those living under less stressful conditions. But does this mean that stress necessarily "causes" mental health woes? Social scientists are embroiled in a long-standing debate referred to as the "selection versus causation" puzzle. The crux of the controversy is whether a stressor such as job loss, poverty, divorce, or difficult caregiving demands causes depression, anxiety, and other mental health conditions, or whether people who are depressed, anxious, or angry are more likely than their healthier counterparts to experience those stressors in the first place.

For example, many studies have found that divorced people have more frequent depression symptoms and drink alcohol more frequently than their married counterparts. Does that mean that the stress of divorce drives people to drink or leaves them heartbroken and emotionally devastated? Perhaps. But another equally plausible explanation is that people who are depressed or who are problem drinkers are more likely to get divorced in the first place; that is, they are "selected" into divorce due to their preexisting problems. Studies show that excessive drinking (especially husbands' drinking) can cause marital strain and, ultimately, marital dissolution. Likewise, research shows that marriage to a depressed partner can be difficult and unrewarding; as such, depressed people are more likely than their

happier counterparts to see their marriages fall apart. If a population-based study shows a statistical association between divorce
and mental health indicators such as depression or substance use,
we cannot necessarily say that divorce "causes" such outcomes.
This is what sociologists mean when they say that "correlation
does not equal causation." Just because two conditions co-occur
does not necessarily mean that one triggers the other. Dozens
of scholarly studies have tried to untangle this vexing puzzle,
and most conclude that that both selection and causation factors
are at play; depression and drinking both increase one's risk of
divorce, but divorce in turn increases symptoms of depression
(especially for women) and frequency of drinking (especially for
men).

Psychosocial Pathways

Sociologists and psychologists propose a range of theories
to explain why and how stress affects mental health, broadly
defined. I provide a brief overview here, as well as examples to
illustrate how stress dampens our emotional health.

ROLE THEORY. Role theory holds that most of our everyday
activities involve carrying out social roles, such as worker or
parent. Each social role is accompanied by a set of expectations
that guide how we carry out our roles. Researchers in the 1970s
were interested in the impact of women's paid employment on
their well-being, especially as women balanced paid work with
demands on the home front. Some scholars believed that juggling multiple roles caused stress for women, and that this juggling act partly accounted for why women are twice as likely as
men to be depressed. Researchers drew attention to the stress
created by simultaneously holding multiple roles that taxed one's
coping resources (role overload) or that were viewed as being in
opposition to one another, such as devoted mother and competent worker (role conflict).

Contemporary research counters that juggling multiple roles is not necessarily stressful, nor does it have uniformly detrimental effects on health. First, recent studies emphasize the salience (or importance) of the role to the individual. Trying to soothe a screaming baby and discipline a surly teenager may be particularly distressing to parents who hold the role of "competent parent" as their most important role in life. Parents who have other salient identities, such as worker or volunteer, may be better equipped to roll with the punches of parenting. Second, multiple roles are most distressing when they are involuntary; as a case in point, surveys have found that for women who wanted to both work for pay and raise children, multiple roles were not particularly distressing. However, full-time mothers who wanted to work for pay or employed women who wanted to be stay-at-home mothers had elevated psychological distress because they felt trapped by their lack of choice. Entrapment, or the feeling that one is stuck in an untenable situation without the capacity to change it, is a powerful predictor of psychological distress.

Researchers have also found evidence for role enhancement processes; those who hold multiple roles may find that stressors in one role are counterbalanced—rather than amplified—by successful experiences in another role. Being passed over for a big work promotion may sting less if one has other roles from which one can derive feelings of competence, such as community volunteer or dedicated friend. Yet the benefits of role accumulation are not universal and reflect structural factors, including access to high-quality and desirable roles. For example, studies of racial differences in stress have found that holding the multiple roles of parent, spouse, and worker provided psychological benefits for whites but not for blacks and Puerto Ricans, due to the poorer-quality jobs held by racial minorities and other work-related stressors, such as discrimination or tokenism.

Role accumulation can also be stress-provoking when people feel that they don't have the time to do all that is expected of them. A recent Gallup Poll found that roughly half of all Americans say that they "do not have enough time" to do what they need to do each day. Of those who reported such time pressures, more than half said that they frequently felt stressed, whereas only 27 percent of persons not operating under time pressures reported feeling stressed. These statistics suggest that it's not necessarily multiple roles that are stressful but the lack of sufficient time to carry out those roles effectively.

CUMULATIVE DISADVANTAGE THEORIES. We've all met someone who just can't catch a break. Take Lynn, a thirty-three-year-old home health aide, for instance. Lynn grew up in a troubled home with emotionally abusive parents. As a result, she struggled with her course work in high school, bounced around different low-paying jobs after graduation, and eventually landed a permanent part-time job caring for sick older adults in their homes. Lynn married young, partly to escape her miserable childhood home. Her rocky marriage lasted just four years before she divorced. Along the way, Lynn battled depression, anxiety, and drinking troubles as she struggled with financial stress and hurtful personal relationships. Lives like Lynn's are not merely a product of bad luck; these difficult lives, marked by multiple chronic and acute stressors, illustrate an important sociological theory called "cumulative disadvantage theory." This perspective proposes that adversity (or stress) gives rise to subsequent adversity, whereas advantage gives rise to advantage. Children like Lynn who grow up in financially and emotionally insecure households often cannot focus on their schoolwork, and thus have poorer grades and lower rates of college attendance, which give rise to less stable professional and family lives in adulthood. These difficulties, in turn, heighten their risk of divorce, job loss, and other mental-health-depleting stressors in adulthood. As such, an event, experience, or characteristic that has adverse effects in the short term may take on increasingly vast implications over time, leading to a greater divide between the "haves" and "have-nots."

Decades of research have shown that people who face more stressors over the course of their lives tend to have poorer mental and physical health; adversities snowball over time, and many people succumb emotionally to the wear and tear. Yet recent research shows that it's not just the accumulation of major events such as deaths and financial insecurity that threaten us. Social scientists using data from daily diary studies such as the National Study of Daily Experience show that our emotional well-being can plummet even when small and nagging microstressors build up throughout the day. A pending work deadline, unpaid bill reminders piling up in the mailbox, sitting in a traffic jam, a burdensome chore, or a spat with a loved one or colleague can add up to symptoms of depression or anxiety.

At first blush, research in the cumulative adversity tradition suggests that people who are beat up by life's difficulties just can't bounce back. That bleak conclusion is not necessarily true. Scholars also have discovered that some individuals are resilient in the face of modest build-ups of adversities, as they develop coping skills or a worldview that helps them to take stress in stride. One recent study tracked more than 2,500 Americans over three years and found a "curvilinear" or upside-down U-shaped association between number of stressors experienced and depression and anxiety symptom levels. People who experienced very high levels of stress and also those experiencing *no stress* fared the worst emotionally. Those who suffered a modest—though not overwhelming—amount of stressors developed coping skills that helped them to deal with new challenges that came their way. Those at the very low end of the stress-exposure curve hadn't developed such skills, whereas those at the very high end of the scale faced multiple adversities that were difficult to overcome, especially given their lack of emotional and financial resources.

However, as we will see in chapter 4, some are more likely to thrive or succumb than others. Subgroups of people, occasionally referred to as "Teflon" and "Velcro," let stress either roll off them or stick to them in harmful ways.

STRESS PROCESS MODELS. The stress process model proposes that most stressors are rooted in social positions that are based, in part, on the characteristics such as age, race, and gender. Exposure to stress is not randomly distributed throughout the population but is highly structured and reflects patterns of inequality. Poor persons tend to be exposed to more stress than wealthier people, whereas blacks and immigrants are more likely than whites and native-born Americans to face stressors related to their social position. A key theme of the stress process model is the launching point of chapter 4—that the impact of stress on health varies widely based on one's other risk factors and resources, such as social support, coping strategies, and economic resources.

For example, discrimination is a persistent stressor that can take a toll on emotional well-being. Those with limited social and economic power are at an elevated risk of experiencing discrimination, and also may have few resources to draw on when managing this stress. Persistent experiences of prejudice and discrimination related to low socioeconomic status, racism, sexism, homophobia, or even body weight (e.g., obesity) require daily adaptations. However, mounting research also shows that while members of historically stigmatized groups may have less social or economic power than others, they may have distinct resources to draw on as they manage stress, including ethnic pride, a sense of solidarity with one's community, close friendships, and an ability to deflect discriminatory experiences as a consequence of others' prejudice rather than one's own shortcomings. These personal resources may help to buffer against the strains that psychiatric epidemiologist Ilan Meyer refers to as "minority stress."

DISCREPANCY THEORIES. Failure and disappointment don't feel good. Although feel-good mantras tell us to pick ourselves up and try again when we fail to achieve a personally important goal, most of us know just how hard that is. Many stressors leave us depressed and anxious because they represent some gap between the "real" and "ideal." Social psychologists dating back to William James have developed different theories that hinge on one key point: you can't always get what you want, and not getting what we want makes us feel bad. Many of the stressors we've already touched on represent some type of discrepancy or gap. At the smallest level of daily hassles, failing to meet a work deadline indicates a gap between what we hoped to do and what we've actually accomplished. Job loss and divorce represent the loss of a desired role or a feeling of failure that one could not sustain a career or a marriage. Even existential strains, such as the realization that one will never achieve their youthful goals of wealth and success, may leave us sad, anxious, or even angry.

Self-discrepancy theory is a useful frame for understanding how gaps between what we want and what we have (or who we are) can compromise our emotional health. Psychologist E. Tory Higgins developed this theory to show how different types of discrepancies affect mental health. He proposed that each of us has an "actual self"—this is who we are. Yet we also have an "ideal self" (who we aspire to be) and an "ought self" (who we feel we should be). Our beliefs about our "ideal" and "ought" selves reflect not only our own hopes and expectations but also our perceptions of what *others* want and expect of us. Each discrepancy leads to particular mental health outcomes. A gap between our "actual" and "ideal" selves leads to sadness over dashed dreams, whereas a discrepancy between "actual" and "ought" may lead to anxiety or guilt about disappointing others.

Discrepancy theories cannot explain all stressors, especially not traumatic ones, yet they do help us to understand strains related to the self and to the many identities we hold.

For example, obesity can be distressing because of the rigid expectations placed on Americans (especially white middle-class women) to maintain a slender physique. Women (even slender women) who perceive a gap between their "actual" and "ideal" weight are at a heightened risk of compromised body image and depressive symptoms, whereas overweight and obese women whose "actual" weight is higher than what their significant others believe they "ought" to weigh are subject to interpersonal mistreatment that may lower their psychological well-being. Threats to one's sense of masculinity may be distressing to men. One fascinating study of prostate cancer patients found that distress levels were highest among men who staunchly believed that men should be strong and virile. Even nonevents, described in chapter 1, can be distressing because they represent a gap between what we are and what we want or expect for ourselves. Sociologists have found that singlehood and childlessness are most distressing for people like Dawn—those who want to reach the milestones of getting married or having a family yet have not done so. By the time people reach old age, most make peace with who they are, yet a minority carry the psychological scars of falling short of their dreams and expectations.

Biological Pathways

In the past decade, biological scientists including neuroscientists and geneticists have generated physiological explanations for why and how social stressors affect our emotional health. Stress affects several physiological systems, including our cardiovascular, endocrine, immune, metabolic, and sympathetic nervous systems. Evidence is much stronger for the biological pathways linking social stressors with physical illness (as we will see in chapter 3), although emerging evidence suggests several plausible biological pathways through which stress affects our mental health. It is important to point out that much of this research has been done on animals or in laboratory settings, and fails to consider all of the complexities of human social life. Still, a brief review of recent research provides provocative insights into the ways that physiological responses to stress may affect our emotional health. I focus briefly on hormonal systems and molecular biology.

STRESS HORMONE PATHWAYS. Stress activates the hypothalamus adrenal axis (HPA) as well as the central nervous system (CNS). When we are in situations that we perceive as being dangerous or distressing, our bodies release stress hormones such as cortisol, dopamine, serotonin, and norepinephrine. When we are in relatively stress-free situations and our chemical systems are working normally, they regulate biological processes such as sleep, appetite, energy, sex drive, and normal moods and emotions. However, when we live under chronically stressful situations, elevated levels of these chemicals may be linked with psychological responses such as depression and anxiety.

Cortisol (also referred to as the "stress hormone") is released in response to stress; in the short term, a spike in cortisol has protective effects for our mind and body because it helps us to survive immediate threats. The release serves as an anti-inflammatory hormone, and increases levels of circulating glucose and energy storage. However, when we live under conditions of constant stress, such as extreme poverty or an abusive marriage, we have prolonged levels of cortisol in the bloodstream, which may elevate our risk of exhaustion, depression, and a range of physical symptoms.

Dopamine (or the "pleasure hormone") levels also are dysregulated in the face of stress, which compromises the ability to feel pleasure, impedes memory and concentration, and creates an inadequate blood flow to the brain. Excessive levels of norepinephrine may trigger anxiety. Serotonin is known as being a "feel-good chemical" that brings us feelings such as joy and enthusiasm. Too much serotonin, however, may produce anxiety, while a deficiency produces poor sleep and exhaustion.

Just as social theories of stress recognize that not all stressors affect our minds and bodies in similar ways, biological studies also reveal that stress does not uniformly make us depressed or anxious. Stressors that are uncontrollable, threaten our physical safety, or that involve trauma tend to generate a cortisol profile consistent with compromised mental health. By contrast, controllable stressors tend to produce a cortisol profile that is associated with better psychological and physical adjustment. Similarly, just as survey-based studies show that the effects of stress tend to decline with time, biological studies show that stress hormone release tends to decline gradually after the onset of an initial stressor occurs.

Researchers recognize, however, that social contexts also shape the ways that stress affects physiological responses and, consequently, our mental health. For example, experiences of workplace discrimination are generally associated with less healthy daily cortisol profiles. A "healthy" or typical cortisol profile is one where levels are highest in the early morning (6 to 8 a.m.), and lowest at midnight. However, one exploration by researchers at the University of Michigan found the least healthy cortisol profiles (i.e., flattest levels of decline throughout the day) among whites who perceived that they were discriminated against, relative to blacks, who evidenced steeper levels of cortisol decline throughout the day. Furthermore, blacks of higher socioeconomic status (SES) showed more harmful (i.e., flatter) daily cortisol profiles than did lower SES blacks. The authors reasoned that blacks, especially those with low levels of education and low-status jobs, might expect mistreatment as part of their daily lives, and thus might be less ruffled by these unjust encounters than their more privileged counterparts.

Although most research on the physiological pathways linking stress to mental health focuses on maladaptive chemical reactions, scientists have recently focused on chemical reactions that may be protective, or that counterbalance the harmful ones.

Oxytocin is a chemical that is released when we have comforting physical contact with a significant other, whether a hug from a friend, or satisfying sexual relations with one's partner. The release of oxytocin, in turn, has a protective effect that counterbalances the health-harming effects of other stress hormones. As we will see in chapter 4, people who have close and supportive relations fare well in the face of stress, because they have both emotional and instrumental help, and they also may experience high levels of the chemical oxytocin, which suppresses other potentially harmful changes in the HPA axis.

MOLECULAR STUDIES. Molecular biologists have recently discovered that stress levels may affect one's corticotropin releasing factor receptor 1 (CRFR1), which in turn affects serotonin receptors (5-HTRs). In short, CRFR1 works to increase the number of 5-HTRs on cell surfaces in the brain, which can cause abnormal brain signaling. Since CRFR1 activation leads to anxiety in response to social and environmental stressors, and 5-HTRs are associated with depression, researchers are beginning to uncover ways that brain processes link stress to anxiety and depression. Although this work is in its nascent stages, scientists are optimistic that drugs may someday be developed to block 5-HTRs that link stress and mental health troubles, thus minimizing the effects of stress on well-being. Likewise, antidepressant medications are now routinely prescribed to regulate HPA axis function, and ultimately lessen some symptoms of depression and anxiety. Critics caution, however, that drugs alone are not sufficient to alter the social situation causing the distress; we will delve into these issues more fully in chapter 5.

In sum, our emotional well-being is powerfully linked to the stressors we face in everyday life. Acute, chronic, and even seemingly insignificant stressors of everyday life may elevate our symptoms of sadness, anxiety and anger, while the death of a loved one is typically accompanied by grief symptoms, and trauma may give rise to post-traumatic stress disorder. The most profound and extreme psychological reaction to stress, suicide, is statistically rare in the United States, but is often an end product of multiple risk factors, including stress, preexisting mental health conditions, substance use, and the means to take one's life. Despite the generally harmful effects of stress, researchers are beginning to document the ways that modest levels of stress can "toughen" people up, help them hone their coping skills, and even promote emotional and spiritual growth following the crisis.

Social scientists have many explanations for how and why stress affects us. Their theories focus on the complex ways that stressors accumulate over time, are based on social characteristics such as race and class, and reflect our feelings of failure (or competence) as we strive to fulfill multiple social roles or achieve the personal goals and expectations we hold for ourselves. Biological scientists, by contrast, focus on the ways that stress triggers chemical and hormonal responses that compromise our emotional well-being. What is clear from theoretical writings and empirical studies is that we should no longer ask the question "Does stress affect mental health?" but rather "When, why, and for whom does stress affect mental health?" As we have begun to see, the effects of stress are neither uniform nor universal, and there is not a "one size fits all" approach to minimizing the harmful effects of stress. We will next delve more fully in the questions of when, why, and for whom stress affects our physical health.

CHAPTER 3

Under Our Skin

HOW AND WHY STRESS AFFECTS OUR PHYSICAL HEALTH

CAN STRESS KILL? POPULAR culture would certainly have us believe so. Classic film buffs may recall the scene from *Now, Voyager* when Charlotte Vale, a quiet spinster who blossoms into a world-traveling sophisticate, has a heated argument with her disapproving mother, who promptly dies of a heart attack. A similar fate struck Horace Giddens in *Little Foxes*. A frail man with a serious heart condition, Horace suffered a heart attack after a vicious spat with his contemptuous wife, Regina. Such dramatic depictions are not limited to the silver screen. On the small screen, *The Simpsons'* Homer Simpson collapsed from a heart attack after his cruel and enraged boss Mr. Burns threatened to fire him from his job at a nuclear power plant.

These melodramatic scenes suggest that stressful encounters may be lethal (often instantaneously), yet we all can think of more gradual or subtle instances in which a friend or family member took ill after a long period of duress. In chapter 1, we met Naomi, who suffered a minor stroke just weeks after the one-two punch of her husband's and mother's deaths. Or Marisol, the twenty-year-old college student who was burning the candle at both ends—working, volunteering, helping her mother with child care, and struggling with a difficult academic course load—before succumbing to the flu during final exams.

Is it really as simple as "shock" or "wear and tear" hurting our hearts and running down our immune systems? Dozens of biological studies document direct linkages between exposure to stress in laboratory settings and physical symptoms such as elevated heart rate, spikes (or drops) in cortisol levels, and susceptibility to colds and infections. Social scientists, by contrast, argue that stress—whether struggles with a daunting college curriculum or the strains of caregiving—is tightly interwoven with other health risks in our lives. As such, it's much harder to conclude that stress alone "causes" our health problems.

Let's suppose that Naomi was a lifelong smoker who upped her habit to two packs a day as a way to calm her nerves during her decade-long stint as a family caregiver. Or that she hadn't gone to the doctor for an annual physical exam in years, because she couldn't take the time away from her round-the-clock caregiving demands. Or that she had lost her health insurance coverage to pay for doctor's visits now that her husband was too ill to work (and the family lost health benefits). Now let's imagine that Marisol slept only four hours a night, and subsisted on energy drinks and sugary cereals, overwhelmed by her college classes and other obligations. Is it really the stressors per se that caused their ailments, or might unhealthy behaviors, lack of time for self-care, or limited access to medical care also have contributed to these women's health woes?

Most stressors do not affect our physical health instantaneously or directly. Rather, stress often is associated with other behaviors and experiences that may compromise our health. A stressor may trigger subsequent changes in our social lives—whether shifts in our relationships, daily routines, or health behaviors—that may threaten our physical health and vigor. In this chapter, I provide an overview of the diverse ways that researchers study the linkages between stress and physical health.

I then review social and biological explanations for why and how stress affects health—whether directly or indirectly. Importantly, no single explanation is sufficient to explain the stress-health connection, because our minds, bodies, and social worlds are interconnected in complex ways.

STRESS AND PHYSICAL HEALTH: HOW DO WE STUDY IT?

Stress is associated with a broad range of health outcomes, including mortality risk and nearly every possible physical symptom or condition, including headaches, heart disease, diabetes, risk of infection, colds, and even how quickly our wounds heal. Most research on the physical health effects of stress relies either on surveys or laboratory designs, although a handful of fascinating studies also rely on chance events or disasters. Each approach sheds light on different aspects of the stress–health connection.

Survey Approaches to Understanding Stress and Health

Survey studies draw on questionnaire data provided by hundreds if not thousands of individuals who report on major stressful events such as divorce or job loss, chronic strains such as caregiving or job stress, and even indicators of early life strains such as exposure to child abuse or poverty. Some surveys include a daily diary component, which asks respondents to report on hassles and uplifts experienced throughout their day for a number of consecutive days or weeks.

Most surveys also obtain extensive measures of self-reported physical health. Rather than directly capturing measures such as current heart rate, most surveys ask people to describe how good their overall health is, with response categories such as excellent, very good, good, fair, or poor. Some surveys obtain detailed illness checklists, which ask respondents to indicate which of a dozen or two health conditions they have been diagnosed with—such as cancer, heart disease, hypertension, or arthritis.

Similarly, symptom checklists capture the number of times in the past week (or sometimes longer) that someone has experienced a dozen or so different health symptoms, ranging from headaches to stomach aches to excessive sweating. Many survey investigators track their research subjects over long periods of time, often until old age. At each follow-up interview, health information is obtained so that researchers can track whether the study participant's health has changed in response to a stressor that occurred between the interviews.

As part of this follow-up, researchers might learn that a participant has died since the last wave of their survey. The investigators may then obtain information on the person's age and cause of death. These data can be obtained from a death certificate; this information helps researchers explore whether people reporting the highest level of stress in surveys are most likely to die prematurely or from particular causes. For example, one study of nearly ninety thousand adults in the United Kingdom found that persons reporting high levels of psychological distress in a survey went on to have higher overall death rates and higher rates of death due to heart disease compared to persons with less stressful lives. Survey studies also may ask about health behaviors, including drinking, smoking, exercise, and diet; health behaviors are an important mechanism that might link stress to health.

Over the past two decades, a growing number of population-based surveys have obtained biological indicators of health (or "biomarkers") in addition to self-reported measures. In such cases, the research team members who administer the survey may also draw blood, obtain a saliva sample, or take a blood pressure reading on their study participants. The most common way to obtain a biological measure today is through the collection of saliva samples; the investigator may ask a research subject to drool into a test tube or to chew on a piece of cotton that absorbs the saliva. Researchers prefer to collect saliva rather than blood because it is less intrusive, meaning that it is less physically and psychologically distressing to research subjects. These newly collected biological data can then be analyzed as another indirect indicator of one's health.

For example, researchers who collect information on a survey participant's blood pressure and other physiological indicators such as cholesterol or the "stress hormone" cortisol can then calculate a person's score on the allostatic load scale. Neurophysiologist Bruce McEwen developed the concept and measure of allostatic load (AL), which refers to a collection of symptoms and conditions that indicate accumulated wear and tear on one's body. Persons who score high on the AL index have been found to have a heightened risk of early mortality and illnesses such as heart disease and diabetes. Thus, this measure helps researchers to understand the ways that physiological responses to chronic stress may hurt one's health and shorten one's life span.

Stress researchers who use survey data and either self-reported health measures or biomarkers typically investigate the long-term or cumulative effects of stress, rather than its immediate and instantaneous effects. For instance, a team of researchers who work on the Midlife Development in the United States (MIDUS) study, a sample survey of more than three thousand adults, found that persons who were poor when growing up (e.g., were on welfare or recalled high levels of financial stress in their families) went on to have higher AL scores in adulthood, compared to their peers who grew up without such financial strain. Another study from the MIDUS found that parents who were raising children with major mental illnesses or developmental conditions such as autism had higher scores on the AL scale. These patterns reveal the long-term "wear and tear" on multiple physiological systems of managing difficult childrearing demands for years on end.

Laboratory-Based Studies of Stress and Health

Surveys can provide us rich information on stressors spanning multiple domains—from work to family to finances—and can capture stressors dating back to our earliest years of life. However, surveys have important limitations, including recall bias. Some survey participants may not be able to accurately recall the distant past, or may even report distorted memories. An adult who is currently depressed may recall their childhood as gray and gloomy, marred by poverty, loneliness, and a lack of emotional support from parents. However, these memories may not reflect the realities of one's childhood, but rather one's current mood state that darkens and alters one's memories.

Another limitation is that it is very difficult to ascertain causation using survey data. A researcher may find a strong correlation (i.e., statistical association) between a recent job loss and headaches, yet there may be other competing explanations for the association. For instance, a worker with persistent debilitating headaches may be frequently absent from work and may be the first to be fired when a boss needs to downsize the company. Social scientists recognize that laboratory-based experiments are the scientific "gold standard" in trying to understand causation. In an experiment, a researcher will typically expose a study participant to a stressor and then measure some biological indicator, such as blood pressure, before and after the stressor. If the indicator changes, then the change can be attributed to the lab-induced stressor. In other cases, the experimenter may randomly assign one half of study participants to a stressful condition and the other half to a neutral condition. If the two groups of study participants then differ on a biological or health outcome, the researcher can plausibly attribute the difference to the stressful condition. Experiments, like surveys, have many shortcomings. They often focus on artificial stressors, such as arguments triggered in the lab, rather than real-world stressors. Still, laboratory-based studies can help us to understand some general principles about stress and health.

The most common approach to inducing stress in a laboratory setting is creating what scientists call a "social evaluative threat." A research subject will perform some task and will then be evaluated publicly by others. For example, one commonly used protocol is the Trier Social Stress Test (TSST). Subjects are required to deliver a public speech in front of a "team of experts" (who often are research staff masquerading as "experts") after having a period of five minutes to prepare. At the end of the speech, the research participants are asked to serially subtract numbers as quickly and accurately as possible. They might be told, "Please start at 100, and count backwards by 7." Each time the participant makes a mistake, he or she is stopped and asked to start over from the initial number. Understandably, we would all be a bit stressed out from giving a public talk and then performing a tricky math exercise in front of a team of so-called experts! The researchers examine whether this stressful experience affects subjects' physical well-being by taking saliva samples when the study respondents first arrive at the lab (i.e., baseline), immediately after the speech and math performance, and then several times afterward.

This study design has been used many times, and consistently shows that salivary cortisol levels show a two- to fourfold increase above one's initial level within a half hour after the stressful lab tasks have been completed. Cortisol, as described in chapter 2, is a stress hormone. Although small increases in cortisol levels can be good for us in the short term by boosting our memory and immune function, persistently high levels are linked with health–depleting physical responses, including suppressed thyroid function, blood sugar imbalances, high blood pressure, lowered immune responses, slowed wound healing, and even a decrease in bone density and muscle tissue. High levels of stress-induced cortisol rises also are linked with abdominal adiposity or "belly fat," which in turn increases our risk of heart attack, stroke, and metabolic syndrome. Although it would be a stretch to say that a stressful lab activity such as doing a math test heightens our risk of heart attack, lab-based studies do provide important insights into the physiological mechanisms linking daily stress and health.

Some skeptical readers may be rolling their eyes, thinking that a math test or public speaking exercise in a laboratory setting doesn't even begin to capture what the real stressors in our lives are like. Rather, the stressors that affect us most may be the ones that are most salient or meaningful to us, such as problems with our marriages, jobs, or health. Lab-based stress researchers, typically psychologists, recognize that more realistic stressors may be a better way to examine linkages between stress and physiological response, and have devised other innovative designs to address these concerns.

One common strategy is for researchers to bring into the laboratory a couple, usually married or in a long-term dating relationship, and then provoke an argument between the partners. A fight with one's long-time love would certainly be more personally salient than would a one-time math exercise. Researchers typically assess the partners' cortisol levels before and after the spat, as a way to track physiological response to stress. In other cases, the investigators may give the subjects a small wound or injection at the beginning of the study, and then examine how quickly the wound heals under the stressful condition of the marital spat.

For example, a team of researchers at Ohio State University brought into their laboratory forty-two healthy married couples, whose ages ranged from twenty to eighty. When the study started, the researchers gave each spouse a small (and relatively painless) cut on his or her forearm. Some study participants were then told to discuss a potentially contentious topic with their spouse, such as in-law woes or financial worries. The researchers found that the couples with the most heated arguments had significantly slower wound healing, evidenced by how quickly the small forearm cut healed. Most subjects healed within five days, but those who had a heated discussion with their spouse took one full day more to heal. The researchers also obtained information on how the couple interacted during the argument. They videotaped the arguments and rated how "hostile" the exchanges were; those couples rated as being hostile toward one another took fully seven days to heal. Taken together, these studies show that an acute stressor, such as a one-time argument, can impair one's immune system, the biological system linked to wound healing. The study also showed that chronic strain, measured as a hostile interactional style between spouses, slowed the healing process even more.

Quasi-Experimental Designs:
Tracking the Health Effects of Chance Events

Skeptical readers, once again, may question whether a lab-induced lovers' spat really qualifies as "stress." Others may question whether experimental designs are adequate to capture major life stressors, such as disaster and trauma. It would clearly be unethical (and impossible) to randomly assign one-half of subjects to a tragic situation, and the other half to a pleasant or neutral situation. However, researchers can sometimes capitalize on "chance events" or unexpected tragedies to explore their impact on physical health. Although these study designs are imperfect and researchers cannot definitively ascertain whether the distressing event "causes" health declines, such studies can provide valuable information on some aspects of health, specifically heart attack risk, in the face of major events.

Extensive international data reveal an increased risk of cardiovascular problems (including heightened blood pressure, heart rate, and heart attack risk) shortly after an earthquake. Earthquakes are unique disasters because they come unexpectedly and suddenly. In addition to the initial stress of the physical destruction, survivors face subsequent chronic stressors, including forced relocation; lack of electricity, water, and telephone service; and decreased access to food. Although psychological distress would certainly increase in such situations, evidence suggests that heart health also suffers. During a 1999 earthquake in Taiwan, twelve people in the local area were already part of a study in which their heart rates were being monitored. The monitors documented that in the minutes before and after the earthquake struck, the subjects' heart rates increased substantially.

Similar patterns were found following the Hanshin-Awaji earthquake Japan in 1995, when blood pressure levels spiked and remained high, even at night when the subjects were sleeping. The number of heart attack patients and subsequent deaths recorded at local hospitals were also detected following the 2004 Central Niigata earthquake in Japan, and the 1994 Northridge, California, quake. However, some earthquakes, such as the 1989 Loma Prieta quake in California, have not been linked with increased risks of heart attack. Researchers point out that there is great variety in the stressfulness of even seemingly devastating events like earthquakes. Some are lower on the Richter scale and less destructive than others, while earthquakes that strike at night are more disruptive and disorienting than those that strike during the day.

Taken together, these survey, laboratory, and chance event studies show that both acute and chronic stressors may trigger physiological responses that are linked to illness risk. Although short-term physical reactions to stress, such as a cortisol spikes, may be adaptive and may help people to flee or adapt to the initial shock, the persistent consequences of stress exposure can be much more severe. As internationally renowned stress researcher Robert Sapolsky has observed, "Stress-related disease emerges, predominantly, out of the fact that we so often activate a physiological system that has evolved for responding to acute emergencies, but we turn it on for months on end, worrying about mortgages, relationships and promotions" (1998).

THE STRESS-HEALTH CONNECTION: SOCIAL SCIENCE EXPLANATIONS

Social scientists, including sociologists, psychologists, and epidemiologists, generally believe that the stress in our daily lives can take a harsh toll on our physical health, even if it takes months or years for these effects to come to fruition. These explanations for *why* stress affects our physical well-being tend to focus on our thoughts, behaviors, emotions, social ties, and social resources—rather than on biology alone. Taken together, social science perspectives suggest that reducing stress in our lives may indeed improve our health, yet it is equally important to repair the social contexts that give rise to stress and to our personal or interpersonal responses to the stress.

Drowning Our Sorrows: The Role of Health Behaviors

A stressful encounter may make our heart race and palms sweat, but stress also makes us behave in ways that hurt (or protect) our health. Think about how you deal when you've had a stressful day at the office, heard bad news, or gone through a heart-wrenching breakup. Do you seek comfort with a glass of wine and a cigarette? Unwind in a yoga class? Work out your frustrations with an invigorating run in the park? Devour a pint of Ben & Jerry's while watching your favorite guilty pleasure reality show? The ways that people alter their behaviors in response to chronic and acute stressors partly explain why some get sick and others don't. Health behaviors, including smoking, alcohol consumption, exercise, eating habits, and drug use, are associated with our risk of illness and death, and play a critical role in linking social stress to physical health.

Most Americans rely on healthy strategies to manage stress. The American Psychological Association (APA) conducts an

annual survey of more than one thousand American adults, and
finds that the most popular strategies for managing stress are listening to music, exercising or taking a walk, spending time with
family and friends, and reading—with more than 40 percent of
Americans using these stress management tactics in 2010.

Yet a significant minority also turns to unhealthy behaviors, such as overeating or eating unhealthy foods (34 percent),
drinking alcohol (19 percent), or smoking (16 percent). The APA
report is consistent with scientific studies showing that stress
is associated with consuming higher-fat diets, eating fast-food
meals, smoking, failed attempts to quit smoking, more frequent
and heavier alcohol use, and skipping exercise. When our nerves
are frayed and our minds are racing with troubling thoughts,
"self-medication" might seem like a sensible and soothing quick
fix. Scientists have documented that nicotine, the addictive drug
component of cigarette smoke, helps to calm people's nerves by
altering activity in parts of the brain that control negative emotions such as anger. Alcohol (in moderation) relaxes or dilates
our blood vessels, and takes the pressure off our hearts. A glass
of wine or a beer also might help us forget our troubles (tem-
porarily) because ethanol, the main psychoactive ingredient in
alcoholic beverages, is a psychoactive drug. After a few drinks,
we experience mild euphoria and loss of inhibition, as alcohol
impairs the regions of the brain that control our actions and
emotions.

Caffeine provides us with a short-term energy boost that
may help us to survive a major work deadline or an intense exam
week. Likewise, sugar is the basic source of energy in the foods
and beverages we consume, so it can give us both energy and
a quick mood lift. The desire to console ourselves with high-
fat "comfort" foods when we're stressed out is perfectly natural,
from an evolutionary perspective. When our bodies are under
constant stress, we physiologically need high-energy foods to
help us persist and weather these challenges. Stress also triggers

hormonal changes that make us crave high-fat, high-salt dishes. Some studies also show that we crave foods such as macaroni and cheese or meatloaf when we're sad, stressed, or anxious because these foods remind us of a more peaceful time or place, when we felt safe, secure, and loved.

While alcohol, cigarettes, sugary or fatty foods, and caffeine might help us to feel better in the short term when we're stressed, in the longer term, these vices may elevate our risk of diseases including heart disease, diabetes, liver disease, high blood pressure, and some cancers. Some health behaviors may create more stress in our lives, which may kick off a vicious circle of taking on even more unhealthy behaviors. Heavy drinkers may have more frequent marital feuds and shakier employment prospects than nondrinkers or abstainers, which in turn may drive them to drink even more. Obesity, which is a consequence of consuming more calories than we burn off through physical activity, increases one's risk of weight-related discrimination and teasing, which in turn may trigger more stress-related eating. While some mood-enhancing behaviors may feel good in the short term, their longer-term health consequences can be dire.

What's more, people who are under the most intense stress also are most likely to turn to unhealthy practices such as smoking, or to say that they're "too busy" or "don't have enough time" to exercise, eat healthy meals, or catch up on their sleep. For example, the 2012 APA study showed that family caregivers were much more likely than noncaregivers to overeat, or to eat unhealthy foods. These behaviors may partly account for family caregivers' elevated risk of heart disease, stroke, and even premature death. One study by Ohio State University researchers Ronald Glaser and Janice Kiecolt-Glaser found that adult children caring for their aged parents with Alzheimer's disease, and mothers caring for terminally ill young children, ultimately died four to eight years younger than their counterparts not providing such care. Ironically, those who provide care for others often lack the time to engage in self-care or other practices that keep them healthy and rejuvenated.

Nudging and Nagging: The Role of Significant Others

Stress drives many people to take on new or ramp up old unhealthy behaviors and eschew healthy ones. While it's easy to blame these self-destructive coping patterns on lack of will-power, that would be an incomplete and inaccurate characterization. Part of the reason why major life stressors such as divorce, widowhood, and unemployment are linked to unhealthy behaviors is that stressed people often lose the significant others or structural supports that helped them to stay healthy, sober, drug-free, or physically fit. Let's consider the case of marriage and marital dissolution. Academic studies show that married people (and especially happily married people) have better physical health and longer lives than their unmarried peers. Yet the health benefits of marriage are larger for men than for women, because women typically play the role of health protector in marriage. Women may nudge their husbands to take their daily medication, eat healthy meals, and curb their drinking. When a marriage ends, whether through death or divorce, a man often loses his helpmate and "nurse."

That's part of the reason why epidemiologic studies show that men are more likely than women to experience downturns in physical health when they divorce or become widowed. Widowers are more likely than married men to die of accidents, alcohol-related deaths, lung cancer, or heart disease during the first six months after their wives die. However, they are no more likely than their married counterparts to die from other causes that are less closely linked to health behaviors, such as stomach cancer or respiratory disease. While romantic movies tell us that widowers may "die of a broken heart" shortly after their wives pass away, due to the stress and emotional drain of the loss, that's only part of the story. Widowers lose not only a lifelong partner but also their wives' reminders to wear a seatbelt, to take their blood pressure medication, and to eat the salad rather than the sixteen-ounce steak for dinner.

Our social ties protect our physical health in another way: social roles such as spouse, worker, and parent impose a sense of obligation, responsibility, and routine into everyday life. These routines and obligations also encourage and promote healthy behaviors. Having a job to report to every morning at 9 a.m. lessens the chances that one will go on an alcohol-frenzied bender the night before. The flip side, however, is that when these roles disappear—whether through job loss, divorce, or death of one's child—the very forces that supported our health behaviors slip away as well. For instance, upon having a child, young men and women who were previously reckless may abandon their "wild" pasts and adopt healthy lifestyles.

Sociologists Deborah Carr, Tetyana Pudrovska, Corinne Reczek, and Debra Umberson (2012) have found that single men who were big drinkers and carousers would give up their evenings at the bar when they married. Their wives would often put their foot down and demand that their husbands grow up, while some men decided on their own that their bar-hopping days were over. Yet when these marriages ended, the men (and some women) cranked up their drug use and drinking, often to dull the pain of the loss or to find emotional support with their old drinking buddies. As Jeffrey, a fifty-seven-year-old divorced participant in the study, said, "As a musician, I guess from the age of sixteen on I was experimenting with drugs . . . marijuana, alcohol, and cocaine. I think after my divorce I went back and just got way in over my head. . . . It didn't really turn to real abuse until after the divorce. It was part of my lifestyle at that time." Although Jeffrey eventually made his way into treatment and got clean, his case vividly shows how the stressful loss of an important role, for instance, being spouse, may trigger a return to one's old self-destructive ways.

A Hard Day's Night: Stress and Sleep

Sleep (or lack thereof) has recently been identified as a critical link between stress and physical health. Sleep problems, which include taking a long time to fall asleep, waking up throughout the night, getting too few hours of sleep, and waking up feeling tired, have been rising steadily in the United States. A 2013 Harris Poll of more than one thousand American adults found that 83 percent say they don't get a good night's sleep on a consistent basis. Severe sleep disorders are less common, but have risen steadily over the past decade. According to the Centers for Disease Control, 10 percent of Americans now have chronic insomnia, and 4 percent have used sleeping medication in the past week. Researchers have recently started to pay greater attention to sleep problems, because inadequate sleep has been linked to the onset and progression of many diseases and health conditions, including diabetes, heart disease, high blood pressure, depression, and abdominal adiposity.

Not all sleep problems are due to stress, of course. Some are due to obesity-related sleep apnea, electronic late-night distractions such as smart phones and 24/7 access to media, a spouse's snoring, a child's nightmares, or an overly energetic pet's desire for nighttime feedings. Yet on the whole, personal and environmental stressors are the most common threats to a good night's sleep. The 2013 Harris Poll found that "stress and anxiety" was the top reason people gave for their sleep problems. Another 47 percent said that they couldn't turn off their anxious thoughts, which caused them to toss and turn or to wake up repeatedly. People who live in unsafe, loud neighborhoods tend to have more difficulty falling asleep and staying asleep, compared to people living in more bucolic and peaceful neighborhoods.

While stress can trigger sleep problems, sleep problems, in turn, can trigger secondary stressors. The vexing cycle of stress and sleep troubles can be difficult to break. Sleep deprivation impairs our performance on complex tasks and compromises our alertness, memory, and ability to think clearly and process information. Not surprisingly, automobile accidents and occupational injuries are linked to sleepiness behind the wheel or on the job. Sleep troubles may also threaten our relationships, either because we're tired, irritable, and may mistreat our loved ones, or because one partner's sleeping patterns may contribute to the other partner's sleep troubles.

For young people today, especially some college students, there's a new wrinkle in the stress–sleep–health cycle: increased reliance on "smart drugs" or "study drugs" such as Adderall and Ritalin. College students, especially those who feel intense pressure to get good grades while juggling other work and extracurricular activities, are turning to "cognitive enhancers." These amphetamine-based drugs, historically prescribed for attention deficit disorder, are now the rage on many college campuses. An estimated 25 percent of students have taken these drugs; the short-term payoff is that the drugs are believed to enhance cognitive function and enable stressed-out students to study for hours with full concentration without getting fatigued. However, scientists have found that these "smart drugs" increase the brain chemical dopamine, raise students' heart rates, and can lead to severe sleep deprivation. The drugs also can be addictive, further contributing to the cycle of school stress, self-medication, and sleep deprivation. Although it's too soon to tell what the long-term consequences are for young people's health, researchers say that at the very least, racing heart rates and sleep deprivation may take a toll in the short term.

The Mind-Body Connection

Chapter 2 described how difficult periods take a toll on our emotional well-being. Yet the mind and the body are closely interconnected, so the psychological reactions we have to stress (such as depression, grief, anxiety, and anger) may in turn affect our physical health. The Buddhist tradition regards the body and the mind as mutually dependent, while folk wisdom tells us that "it's not what you eat, it's what's eating you" that makes people ill. Scientific evidence, too, shows that the mind and the body are mutually influential. At the most basic level, persons who are depressed and have a difficult time getting motivated may be less likely to engage in protective health behaviors, to sleep regularly, to seek out medical care when needed, or to engage in self-care. Mental health symptoms such as anger, hostility, or withdrawal from others may build a barrier between the stressed-out individuals and the friends and family who could help them to work through their stress.

Emerging scholarship argues that mental health conditions, especially depression, can "cause" physical health conditions. For example, the American Psychological Association (2007) recently published a report titled *Contributions Toward Evidence-Based Psychocardiology*, which emphasized how depression and hostility could contribute to heart disease by increasing stress hormones. However, most researchers find two other arguments are far more plausible. First, if risk of depression and chronic illness are correlated, it's more likely that the depression is a result—rather than the cause—of the chronic illness. Health psychologist Howard Leventhal and colleagues have found that the tasks of managing one's illness, whether regularly seeking treatments, altering one's diet and lifestyle, or giving up vigorous activities one once liked to do, may depress one's mood.

Second, if depression and chronic illness co-occur, it's possible that the association is spurious. That is, both conditions may result from a shared set of triggers, such as persistent poverty that makes one feel consistently demoralized and hopeless yet at the same time prevents one from eating healthy foods, buying a gym membership, paying for hypertension medications, or seeing regular care from a personal physician—all of which may conspire to increase one's risk of heart disease. No one would refute that problems of the mind and of the body are closely intertwined, yet there is far less agreement about which came first. However, most scholars recognize that many stress-related physical and mental health concerns are deeply rooted in social and economic inequalities.

Social Class: The Fundamental Cause behind the Stress-Health Link?

One of the most well-established findings in epidemiological studies is the "social class gradient" in health. Regardless of what health outcome is considered, including frequency of headaches, muscle pain, diabetes risk, cancer, disability, or death, those with fewer social and economic resources fare worse than those with richer resources. The social class gradient in health may partly explain the linkage between stress and physical health; as sociologist Leonard Pearlin's stress process model tells us, not all people are equally likely to be exposed to stress. Those possessing the fewest social and economic resources, whether education, wealth, income, occupational status, or a safe and secure living space, are at the greatest risk of just about every work-, family-, and social-network-related stressor, and these stressors in turn may compromise health.

Sociologists Bruce Link and Jo Phelan (2010) developed fundamental cause theory (FCT) to explain the steep social class gradient in health. Social-class-based disparities in physical health are stark; for example, people at the top of the income ladder in the United States live seven years longer, on average, than those on the lower rungs. Fundamental cause theory argues that these stark health disparities exist because social class encompasses a sweeping array of resources, including money, knowledge, power, and beneficial social connections that may affect health in powerful ways. The uneven distribution of stress throughout the social hierarchy contributes to the class gradient in health. Lower socioeconomic status (SES) increases one's risk of stressful life events, ranging from divorce to job loss to crime victimization, and one's chronic stressors, including poor, overcrowded and unsanitary living conditions; persistent economic strain; and discrimination. Social class also is associated with having fewer coping resources, including supportive social ties, effective problem-solving strategies, and the financial means to escape a distressing situation.

One study by epidemiologist Sandro Galea and colleagues examined social factors related to adult mortality from 1980 to 2007; some of the most "lethal" social factors they identified sit at the intersection of poverty and stress. They estimated that 133,000 deaths in the United States in 2000 could be attributed to poverty, and that a whopping 176,000 deaths could be blamed on racial segregation, whereas car accidents accounted for just 119,000 deaths. Of course, it is difficult to prove the bold claim that the stress of living in a racially segregated, poor, or social isolated neighborhood will "kill." However, scholars working in the tradition of fundamental cause theory draw our attention to the ways that stress and economic inequality are inextricably tied, and to how the two adversities heighten one's risk of multiple physical and mental health woes.

THE STRESS-HEALTH CONNECTION: PHYSIOLOGICAL PATHWAYS

Our social environments and resources clearly contribute to the stress-health link. Yet since the 1980s, many scientists have started to cast a spotlight on biological rather than social explanations for the stress-health connection. In the past three decades, a tidal wave of articles has been published on the biological pathways linking stress to health. This rise is due, in part, to technological advances in how efficiently we can measure physiological responses to stress. Scientists working in the fields of psychoneuroimmunology are better equipped than ever before to evaluate the brain's responses to stress, while biological scientists can quickly measure and assess physiological responses in heart rate, cortisol levels, and breathing. While this explosion of scholarship is new, it shares its fundamental roots with the earliest research on stress, conducted by endocrinologist Hans Selye.

Early Writings of Selye

Selye viewed physical distress as an automatic response to any environmental stressor. In response to stress, the body would pass through the three distinct stages of alarm, resistance, and exhaustion. In the alarm stage, the autonomic nervous system is stimulated, sympathetic nervous system activity is suppressed, and muscle tone decreases. In the resistance stage, the body tries to maintain a high level of functioning in order to survive the threat. In the final exhaustion stage, endocrine activity is heightened, and high levels of cortisol start to take their toll on the body's circulatory, digestive, immune, and cardiovascular systems. Human energy and resources are depleted, and permanent damage to the body might result from the cumulative wear and tear.

In the six decades since the publication of Selye's path-breaking work, scientists working in fields ranging from genetics to psychophysiology to neuroscience have elaborated on the biological pathways linking stress to physical health conditions. While Selye assumed that all stressors affect physical functioning, contemporary research sheds light on why some health conditions, especially heart disease, are susceptible to particular types of stressors. A full explication of the physiological pathways linking stress to health is complicated and beyond the scope of this slim book; however, in the next few paragraphs I provide a brief overview of the ways that key biological systems, including the central nervous, cardiovascular, and immune systems, respond to stress, and how these responses may carry long-term implications for our risk of disease and death.

Physiological responses to stress involve the direct stimulation of the central nervous system (CNS) and a hormonal relay system among three organs: the adrenal glands, located at the top of each kidney; the hypothalamus; and the pituitary gland, located in the brain. Both the CNS and the hypothalamic-pituitary-adrenal (HPA) axis play a critical role in linking stress with physical health. Most research on social stress and health has focused on the cardiovascular and immune systems because they are closely related to the progression of common diseases, including heart disease, stroke, and pneumonia.

Stress and Cardiovascular Health

Stress researchers are particularly concerned about heart disease because it is the leading cause of death in the United States and in most wealthy developed nations today. Of the roughly 2.5 million deaths in the United States in 2010, about 600,000 were due to heart disease. Stress is clearly implicated as a risk factor for heart disease and stroke—although the association may not be as direct as films like *Now, Voyager* might lead us to believe. Our personal reactions to stress account in large part for the stress-heart disease link. High stress reactivity increases vascular inflammation, which leads to a buildup of plaque in our arteries (i.e., atherosclerosis). When our arteries are "clogged" with plaque buildup, our blood flows less freely and increases our risk of myocardial infarction (i.e., heart attack) and stroke. Stress and stress reactivity also increase our production of platelets. Platelets are a type of blood cell, and their main purpose is to prevent us from bleeding. Platelet activation releases substances into the blood stream that adhere to (or "stick to") our arteries, which leads to plaque buildup; as such, it may contribute to our risk of heart disease.

Evidence linking stress to heart disease is compelling and abundant. The INTERHEART study, a study of psychosocial stress and heart attack risk among twenty-five thousand people in fifty-two countries, found that people who reported "permanent" stress at work or home had roughly twice the risk of developing an MI (myocardial infarction) compared to those who did not experience comparable stress. These effects were generally consistent across geographic regions, by ethnicity, and gender. Studies have also identified particular stressors that are especially closely tied to heart disease. One stressful aspect of work—facing high demands but having little control over one's work environment—is a widely documented predictor of heart troubles, including high blood pressure. Working under relentless time pressures is highly distressing, as we all know. However, the pressure to get our work done while having little control over when, how, and with whom we do our work is a particularly devastating combination. Yet not all people are equally likely to develop heart disease in the face of stress. As we will see in chapter 4, those with the highest levels of stress reactivity, or who respond strongly to stress, are more likely to develop heart disease in the face of stress.

Stress and Immune Function

Marisol, the overworked and exhausted college student we met earlier in this book, fell sick with the flu after juggling multiple school, family, and work activities. One explanation for Marisol's plight is that her immune system succumbed to the chronic stressors in her life. The immune system protects our bodies from foreign materials, such as viruses and bacteria, by releasing into our circulatory system both white blood cells and antibodies. (An antibody is a protein produced by the body's immune system when it detects harmful substances.) When we're under extreme stress, as Marisol was, our immune responses falter, making the body less able to defend itself against harmful foreign materials.

Stress increases our risk of viral infections such as the flu and colds. Most of this evidence comes from laboratory studies, similar to the ones described earlier in this chapter. In studies of the immune system, researchers typically ask healthy volunteers to answer questions about the stress in their lives, and then inoculate them with a virus. Researchers typically track their subjects for several days, and find that those subjects who had been exposed to the highest levels of stress—whether reported on their questionnaires or induced in the lab (such as a math test)—showed evidence of increased susceptibility to upper respiratory infection.

Recent work on stress and immune function further shows that cortisol plays a critical role in the stress-infection link. Stress researcher and psychologist Sheldon Cohen has conducted many studies showing how we get common colds after bouts of stress. His work shows that prolonged exposure to stress lessens our immune cells' capacities to respond to hormonal signals that normally regulate inflammation. In turn, those with the inability to regulate the inflammatory response are more likely to develop colds when exposed to a virus. It's not just colds that we're at risk of, however. Inflammation plays a role in many diseases, such as cardiovascular, asthma and autoimmune disorders.

Mounting research also shows that stressors dating back to our earliest years may have powerful long-term effects on inflammation and ultimately on our disease risk. Adults who had been the victims of psychological, sexual, or physical abuse in childhood or who grew up with a problem-drinker parent have elevated levels of three body chemicals that are markers of inflammation: interlukin-6 (IL-6), C-reactive protein (CRP), and fibrinogen. Children who grew up in impoverished households also show higher levels of persistent and multiple infections over the life course. While the bulk of evidence suggests that the wear and tear of multiple stressors and cumulative adversities under-mine our immune function, some scholars have recently posited that some young people growing up under conditions of stress and adversity may be particularly resilient in the case of infec-tion. Likewise, children who grow up in relatively stress-free and peaceful environments may not "toughen up" to illness or infec-tion. The "hygiene hypothesis" holds that those who face few pathogenic challenges in early life may have poorly regulated inflammatory and immune responses later in life. Although evidence is preliminary, such findings are provocative in that they provide evidence of resilience in the face of adversity, a topic we will delve into more fully in chapter 4.

In sum, scientists working in a range of different methods and disciplines agree that stress takes a toll on our physical well-being, although experts vary in how much stock they place in social versus biological explanations for the stress-health link. Most scientists recognize, however, that we need to pay careful attention to both social and biological pathways if we really want to understand human health and well-being. Answering the questions of why and how stress affects health is the first critical step on the path to interventions and solutions. As chapter 5 will show, scientists' theories and empirical findings help us to figure out whether the best way to protect against stress-related health woes is through prescribing a medication, offering medical care and counseling, or altering the social structure that gives rise to health-depleting stressors.

CHAPTER 4

Why Some Crumble and Others Bounce Back

RISK AND RESILIENCE IN THE FACE OF STRESS

CALVIN, THE MARRIED FATHER of two sons, is a talented computer programmer and math whiz who can't hold down a job. A thirty-five-year-old college graduate with a quirky and occasionally off-putting sense of humor, Calvin lost his most recent job as a programmer at a high-tech firm because he regularly dropped the ball on tasks his boss needed done ASAP. Rather than bucking up and vowing to do better on those occasions when his boss scolded him, Calvin would grow more agitated, anxious, and disorganized. He would fall short on his work tasks, hide his mistakes from others, and couldn't develop a plan for winning back the support and respect of his coworkers. "Why bother," he'd lament, assuming that he was bound to fail and disappoint. Calvin would unwind each night by smoking a joint, trying to block out memories of his stressful day at the office. After he let down his boss one final time, Calvin was fired. More than two years later, he is still unemployed. Too despondent to exercise and relying on food to uplift his mood, Calvin has gained weight and developed early-onset diabetes.

He spends most of the day distracting himself with video games and Facebook. Although he half-heartedly looks for work, he has applied for only a handful of jobs, assuming that he doesn't have a chance. His inability to get his life back on track and his persistent health woes have placed strains on his marriage. His long-suffering wife, Keshia, a high school teacher, is tired of supporting him emotionally and financially, creating even more stress and feelings of inadequacy for Calvin.

Contrast Calvin's situation with that of Marcus, also a thirty-five-year-old married father of two children. An analyst and statistician in the volatile industry of finance, Marcus has switched jobs four times in as many years. Twice, he quit because he found the commute and daily tasks to be unappealing. He was fired once because his work approach and personality were a "bad fit" for the new employer, and was laid off once when the start-up he worked for folded. Marcus always lands on his feet, though, quickly securing new work. Between jobs, he'd network at professional association events, reach out to former colleagues using social media, tirelessly sift through online job listings, and read up on the latest financial industry news—all the while retaining his gregarious personality and engaging sense of humor. Although he worried about supporting his wife, Sheryl, a nurse, and two young daughters during his brief stints of unemployment, Marcus remained optimistic that things would resolve successfully. On those days when he felt anxious about his job prospects, he worked through those worries on early morning jogs through his neighborhood.

At first blush, Calvin and Marcus are very similar. Both are college-educated fathers and husbands who work in highly technical and competitive fields. Both lost their jobs against the backdrop of a recession, when hopes of finding new work were slim. Yet the two managed their work stressors and subsequent job searches in entirely different ways. Calvin broke under the pressure of a stressful work environment and subsequent layoff, whereas Marcus rebounded quickly. Why do some people bounce back from—and even thrive—in the face of stress and challenge, whereas others are devastated by it? Researchers recognize that even a single stressor (such as job loss) can affect two people in very different ways. The characteristics that buffer against or intensify the health-depleting stress are referred to as moderators. Dozens of psychological, demographic, interpersonal, biological, and structural factors may intensify or mollify the effects of stress on health. I focus on two main psychological factors (coping strategies and personality), four demographic characteristics (age, sex, race/ethnicity, and socioeconomic status), one interpersonal resource (social support), and one set of biological factors (genetic phenotypes) that have been implicated as a pivotal link in the stress-health equation.

PSYCHOLOGICAL INFLUENCES

Coping Strategies

"Coping" refers to our efforts to ward off or manage a stressful situation, and our efforts to minimize the distress that results from these experiences. Our coping strategies typically fall into one of two broad categories: problem-focused or emotion-focused. Researchers typically document a person's coping style by asking a series of questions about how one usually deals when they have problems. For example, figure 4.1 shows items from the Brief COPE, an inventory designed to identify the specific ways people deal with their problems. Although most people use different strategies to cope with different problems, we also have general tendencies to favor one class of strategies over the other.

Problem-focused coping (PFC) is directed at the stressor itself; we might take steps to avoid or remove the stressor, or to reduce its impact on our lives in those situations where we can't make the stressor disappear. If our workplace is downsizing and we know that a layoff is imminent, we might save money, cut

FIGURE 4.1
Examples of Common Coping Strategies

Coping Strategy	Specific Examples
Self-Distraction	I turn to work or other activities to take my mind off things.
	I do something to think about it less, such as going to movies, watching TV, reading, daydreaming, sleeping or shopping.
Active Coping	I concentrate my efforts on doing something about the situation I'm in.
	I take action to try to make the situation better.
Denial	I say to myself 'this isn't real.'
	I refuse to believe that it has happened.
Substance Use	I use drugs or alcohol to make myself feel better.
	I use drugs or alcohol to help me get through it.
Use of Emotional Support	I get emotional support from others.
	I get comfort and understanding from someone.
Use of Instrumental Support	I get help and advice from other people.
	I try to get advice or help from other people about what to do.
Disengagement	I give up trying to deal with it.
	I give up the attempt to cope.
Venting	I say things to let my unpleasant feelings escape.
	I express my negative feelings.
Positive Reframing	I try to see it in a different light, to make it seem more positive.
	I look for something good in what is happening.
Planning	I try to come up with a strategy about what to do.
	I think hard about what steps to take.
Humor	I make jokes about it.
	I make fun of the situation.
Acceptance	I accept the reality of the fact that it has happened.
	I learn to live with it.
Religion	I try to find comfort in my religion or spiritual beliefs.
	I pray or meditate.
Self-Blame	I criticize myself.
	I blame myself for things that happened.

SOURCE: Carver, C. S. (1997). You want to measure coping but your protocol's too long: Consider the Brief COPE. *International Journal of Behavioral Medicine, 4,* 92–100.

back on our spending, apply to many other jobs, learn a new skill, or work hard at our current job so that we're indispensable to our boss. We tend to use PFC when we see our situation as something we can change or improve. For instance, even after Marcus lost his job, he kept up his knowledge of the financial industry, relied on social contacts, and pounded the pavement to find work.

Emotion-focused coping (EFC), conversely, focuses on allaying our emotional or physical distress when faced with a difficult situation. We tend to use EFC strategies when we believe that nothing can be done to alter our unfortunate situation. Emotion-focused coping encompasses a broad range of strategies; productive ones include expressing our negative emotions (e.g., yelling or crying), soothing our negative feelings (e.g., relaxation techniques, seeking emotional support), finding humor in the situation, or even turning to prayer. However, other EFC tactics impede us from overcoming the stressful situation and may actually worsen it, such as dwelling on our negative thoughts (e.g., rumination), or passive attempts to escape the situation, such as denial, avoidance, and even fantasizing. Calvin exemplified such maladaptive EFC responses to stress; by lighting up a joint to forget about his stressful work day, Calvin simply made himself groggy and inefficient at work the following day, perpetuating his professional troubles.

Rumination, or continually replaying the negative event in our minds and stewing in our own sadness, is a particularly harmful response to stress, according to late psychologist Susan Nolen-Hoeksema. Ruminators prolong their feelings of sadness and loneliness by dwelling on them, and may even intensify their anxiety by fixating on all the things they feel they did wrong. In short, ruminators just can't "get over it." New evidence suggests that ruminating may even affect physiological functioning, and ultimately our physical health. In one recent study, a team of researchers brought young women into a laboratory setting, and asked each of them to give a speech explaining why they would be an ideal candidate for a job opening. Their audience consisted of two stern "interviewers" wearing white coats, sitting stone-faced at a nearby table. Although these two interviewers were really study confederates, the young women genuinely believed that the curmudgeons were potential bosses. After giving the speech under clearly nerve-wracking conditions, half of the women were asked to think about their underwhelming performance in the job interview, whereas the other half were asked to think about neutral or pleasant topics such as shopping. Researchers took blood samples from the women before and after the stressful speech, and found that C-reactive protein (CRP) levels were considerably higher among those who were asked to dwell on their speech. Among the ruminators, CRP levels continued to rise for at least one hour after their speech. By contrast, among the women who thought about neutral topics, CRP levels returned quickly to their prestressful event levels. As noted in chapter 3, CRP is an indicator of inflammation and is associated with one's risk of illness and infection.

Clearly, ruminating is an unhealthy coping tactic. In general, PFC strategies are considered more effective than EFC strategies. Problem-focused coping is associated with lower levels of psychological distress in the face of life's adversities, whereas emotion-focused coping is linked to higher levels of sadness, worry, and hopelessness. Many specific tactics encompassed under EFC are considered "disengagement coping," or passive responses geared toward forgetting or blocking out the stressor. This disengagement hurts one's chances of recovery from the stressor. For instance, research shows that patients with health problems—ranging from cancer to dental troubles—who relied on avoidance tactics, such as denying that they were ill, deteriorated more quickly than those who faced up to their problems. The latter group devised ways to tackle their symptoms (e.g., getting treatment) and minimize their distress (e.g., seeking emotional support from friends). Effective PFC may even heighten psychological well-being, by fostering a sense of mastery, efficacy, and accomplishment. However, there are rare instances in which EFC may be better for us than PFC. Problem-focused coping is ineffective when we're suffering an irreversible and irreplaceable loss, such as the death of one's spouse or child. We can't bring our spouse back to life, but we can soothe our grief by turning to friends for social support, distracting ourselves with happy memories of our late spouse, or finding meaning (or even humor) in the situation.

In sum, how we cope with stress partly determines whether we'll thrive mentally and physically, or succumb to adversity. But coping strategies are not the only factors that explain why some bend, some break, and others bounce back. Other psychological factors, especially personality, also matter. Our personalities partially dictate whether we cope actively or passively, successfully or unsuccessfully.

You've Got Personality: Which Traits Are Protective?

"You've got personality" sounds like a terrific compliment; it means that people view us as fun, upbeat, and pleasant to be around. Likewise, when Americans are asked to name the most desirable trait is in a romantic partner, the most popular answer is typically "good personality" (tied with "honesty"), while good looks and money are much further down the list. But what is a "good" personality? And how does it relate to stress?

Personality refers to our enduring emotional or temperamental traits; some of us are low-key, while others are intense and competitive. These traits are partly genetic, partly a product of how we were raised as children, and partly an outcome of formative experiences throughout our lives. Our personalities may change slightly with age; most of us are more confident and outgoing as adults than we were as awkward teens. Workplace obligations often make us more conscientious, while taking on roles such as parent, spouse, or caregiver to aging parents may make us more nurturing and compassionate. Likewise, our personalities may change slightly in different settings; we may be warm and funny with friends, yet more serious and rigid with coworkers. On the whole, though, how outgoing, cynical, nervous, or cheerful we are relative to other people stays fairly constant over time and across settings. The personality traits we possess (or lack) are an important resource (or liability) when it comes to dealing with stress. Some become flustered and angry when they misplace their car keys, whereas others keep a stiff upper lip and a level head even when they're in the throes of military combat.

Personality affects whether we experience a stressful situation, the extent to which we view a particular event or experience as stressful, our selection of a particular coping strategy, and how effectively we employ this coping strategy. Personality researchers, typically psychologists by training, have developed dozens of inventories that measure and assess our personality traits. I focus on three personality measures that are considered particularly important for understanding our reactions to stress: Type A versus Type B; optimism versus pessimism; and attributes of the Big 5 personality scale.

TYPE A VERSUS TYPE B. Early research suggested that there were two main personality types that differ starkly in how they respond to stress. Type As are tightly wound, competitive, and intense. They perpetually feel a sense of time urgency—walking and talking quickly, getting frustrated while waiting for an elevator, and checking their watch every ten seconds for fear of being late to their next appointment. Type As also score high on the personality trait of hostility, or becoming angry, upset, and even aggressive when things don't go their way. Type Bs, by contrast, are more relaxed and better able to roll with life's punches. In general, Type Bs tend to have better overall health than Type As; their laid-back approach to life allows them to

handle stress without cracking under the pressure. This equanimity translates into a higher quality of life, better emotional
well-being, lower risk of heart disease, and less duress on one's
immune and gastrointestinal systems.

The two personality types also manage stress in different
ways. Type As are more likely to pursue challenge—climbing
mountains rather than napping on mountainsides, as the cartoon
in figure 4.2 suggests. They may also gravitate toward situations
that are inherently stressful, such as deadline-intensive competitive jobs or romantic partners with a combative streak. Type As
who invest their time and energy more heavily in work challenges than in personal relationships are prone to social isolation,
a major risk factor for poor health. Type Bs are more likely than
Type As to seek and welcome support from others during their
time of distress; social support is among the most effective buf-
fers against the health-depleting effects of stress. Type As may
also find that their natural intensity and competitive spirit can
be heightened by situational stress; a person who feels constant
time pressure will be even more stressed when faced with work
deadlines, financial pressures, or work-family demands.

OPTIMISM VERSUS PESSIMISM. Winston Churchill famously pro-
claimed, "The pessimist sees difficulty in every opportunity. The
optimist sees the opportunity in every difficulty." Churchill's words
mesh closely with laypersons' notions of optimists, who "view the
glass as half-full," while their pessimistic counterparts "view the
glass as half-empty." Optimists and pessimists also approach stress
and challenge in different ways. Optimists, like financial analyst
Marcus, possess great confidence that they can overcome the
stressors in their path, while pessimists like Calvin tend to be filled
with doubt about both their own capacities to overcome hurdles,
and the likelihood that their situation will ever change for the better. The former, not surprisingly, is more closely linked to effective
(and health-enhancing) problem solving.

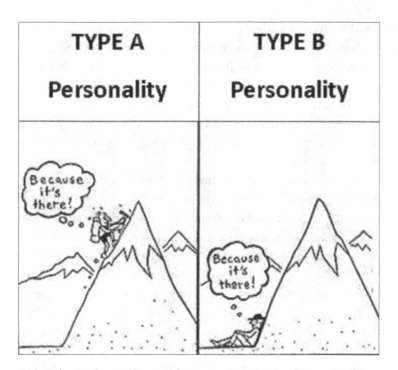

4.2. What's the Difference between Type A and Type B?

How one copes is shaped, in part, by traits such as optimism and pessimism. One theory of how we manage stress is called "expectancy-value theory." This perspective says that our success in meeting our goals depends on two main factors: our evaluation of how much we want to meet our goal (that is, how desirable or undesirable the goal is), and our sense of confidence that we can successfully attain it. Let's say that we lose our job and the thing we want most is a new job. Most people might agree that a new job is highly desirable, even necessary, and something we should pursue with zeal. Yet the extent to which we pursue that job hinges on how likely it is that we think we'll get it. An optimist like Marcus approaches such challenges with self-assuredness and hope ("Someone has got to get the position; it might as well be me!"), whereas a pessimist like Calvin sees his chances as dim ("I'll never get the job, so why bother applying?"). This confidence pushes the optimist to cope proactively, which is linked to better health. Studies show that cancer patients who are optimistic have better survival outcomes, in part, because they seek out social support, are more vigilant about getting effective medical care, may comply with doctors' recommendations, and may find meaning and purpose even in the face of health threats.

Not all researchers agree that optimists deal with stress more effectively, however, or that optimists fare better in the face of threat. Barbara Ehrenreich, author of *Bright-Sided: How Positive Thinking Is Undermining America*, argues that Americans' emphasis on optimism dupes people into believing that simply "thinking positive thoughts" will melt away our stressors and cure our health woes. Rather, Ehrenreich notes, some people are optimistic precisely because everything has gone their way in life; they have the money, friendships, good jobs, comfortable homes, and other resources that predispose them to health and happiness. These fortunate people would fare just fine even if they did not possess perpetually sunny outlooks. By focusing on fixing one's temperament rather than repairing the social inequalities that generated the stressor in the first place, practitioners and policy makers are neglecting the real root of stress and its accompanying health effects, says Ehrenreich.

A handful of scholars even suggest that optimism taken to the extreme (called "unrealistic optimism") is associated with ineffective coping. Dreamy-eyed Pollyannas may underestimate their risk of a stressor such as job loss or divorce, and do not take adequate steps to prepare. Likewise, those who are overly optimistic about their health may turn a blind and blithe eye to potentially dangerous symptoms, or may engage in unhealthy behaviors because they can't foresee a downside of doing so. For instance, smokers with unrealistically high levels of optimism are less likely than their pessimistic counterparts to quit smoking, while highly optimistic college students underestimate their chances of developing drinking problems and then experience more alcohol-related woes such as hangovers or missed classes. Those who are more pessimistic, by contrast, engage in more proactive coping to forestall what they see as quite realistic and likely consequences of drinking. In sum, while optimists generally cope better than pessimists, a rosy outlook—taken to the extreme—can prevent productive actions.

BIG FIVE. Most Americans have heard of Type A and Type B personalities, and nearly all know the difference between an optimist and a pessimist. However, they may not know that one of the most widely used measures of personality is called the "five factor model," which encompasses the traits of neuroticism, extraversion, openness to experience, agreeableness, and consciousness. According to Oliver John, who designed the Big Five personality scale, these traits are associated with how people cope with stress, and consequently help us to understand why some fall ill in the face of stress, whereas others can weather such storms easily. (See figure 4.3 for traits capturing each of the five attributes.)

Neuroticism is one of the most frequently studied personality traits in the stress literature. People high in neuroticism are prone to emotional distress, depressive symptoms, anxiety, somatic complaints, and negative mood, and are likely to view the world around them as stressful and unsafe, often conjuring up mental images that are far worse than reality. The classic neurotic personality type is Woody Allen's film character Alvy Singer. Singer, the antihero of *Annie Hall*, spent his childhood worrying that the universe was going to explode, while in adulthood his exaggerated worries about everything from sex to political conspiracies to anti-Semitism threatened his romantic relationships. Off the silver screen, highly neurotic people tend to alienate those friends and family members who can help them

FIGURE 4.3
Dimensions of the Big 5 Personality Scale

Dimension	Low Scorers	High Scorers
Extraversion	Loner	Joiner
	Quiet	Talkative
	Passive	Active
	Reserved	Affectionate
Agreeableness	Suspicious	Trusting
	Critical	Lenient
	Ruthless	Soft-hearted
	Irritable	Good-natured
Conscientiousness	Negligent	Conscientious
	Lazy	Hard-working
	Disorganized	Well-organized
	Late	Punctual
Neuroticism	Calm	Worried
	Even-tempered	Temperamental
	Comfortable	Self-conscious
	Unemotional	Emotional
Openness to experience	Down-to-earth	Imaginative
	Uncreative	Creative
	Conventional	Original
	Uncurious	Curious

To evaluate your own scores on the Big Five scale, please see http://www
.outofservice.com/bigfive/

cope with stress, and their exaggerated worries derail them from devising sensible solutions to the stressors they face. People high in neuroticism often rely on the least effective EFC strategies, such as wishful thinking, escapist fantasy, self-blame, withdrawal, and passivity. Neurotics like Calvin also tend to hide from their troubles, turning to unhealthy forms of denial such as alcohol or drug use. Some neurotics also carry around anger and hostility, and are at greater risk of cardiovascular disease and slower recovery from illness when faced with insurmountable stressors.

Extraverts tend to have outgoing and optimistic personalities and are sociable, carefree, and proactive in their activities and relationships. Those high in extraversion enjoy spending time with people, an attribute that benefits them in times of stress. Introverts are at the opposite end of the spectrum, and are quieter, more thoughtful, controlled, and careful. They tend to withdraw socially after a stressful encounter, which exacerbates the harmful consequences of the stress. For these reasons, extraverts tend to have better physical and mental health than introverts, including lower levels of depression, anxiety, suicidal ideation, and eating disorders. Extraverts also tend to rely on PFC approaches—developing constructive ways to overcome stress and shifting their mindset to minimize the emotional distress linked to the stressor.

Agreeableness is closely related to yet distinct from extraversion. Agreeableness encompasses traits that foster close and rewarding relationships with others, including being friendly, helpful, empathetic, and able to keep one's negative feelings in check. Agreeable people tend to have less stress in their lives, if only because they tend to find themselves in (or consciously create) situations marked by low levels of interpersonal conflict and stress. They also tend to become less upset by others' misbehavior than their less agreeable counterparts, thus dulling the effect of stressors such as marital strain on health and well-being. Agreeableness is associated with help seeking, problem solving, and positive reappraisal, and lower levels of reliance on avoidant and ruminative EFC strategies. As we saw in the case of Marcus, the ability to maintain a positive outlook and sustain warm friendships during times of stress is a key element in adapting to strains such as persistent unemployment.

Conscientious people tend to be reliable, hard-working, future-oriented, and self-disciplined—often turning their noses up at impulsive or reckless behavior. These level-headed people are particularly effective at coping because they anticipate and plan for predictable stressors. For instance, they may prepare financially for a spouse's eventual death and thus do not face the same financial distress that other widows or widowers face. Conscientious people also tend to avoid irrational actions that can compromise their health or well-being. Not surprisingly, they enjoy longer life spans than their less diligent counterparts, in part because they have fewer high-risk behaviors and are more compliant with doctors' orders. A further benefit of conscientiousness is that these people carry great confidence that they can handle future stressors, given their past record of success. As a result, they tend to employ active strategies for managing stress, relying on tactics such as seeking support, proactive problem solving, and cognitive restructuring—and avoiding passive techniques such as denial, substance use, and dwelling on negative emotions.

The fifth factor, openness to experience, encompasses curiosity, open-mindedness, flexibility, and tolerance for novel ideas and situations. Although stress researchers have paid less attention to openness than to the other four factors, some studies suggest that individuals who are open to experience tend to use humor when dealing with stress, and are particularly creative problem solvers. Openness is distinct from the other four scales, however, in that it is closely tied to one's level of education. As we will see later, education is an important coping resource because it is linked not only to thoughtful and creative problem solving but also with having the economic resources to seek out support and to restructure one's stressful environment.

DEMOGRAPHIC FACTORS

The types of stressors we experience, the resources we have to deal with them, and their effects on our health and well-being are closely tied to our social and demographic characteristics, such as age, sex, race or ethnicity, and socioeconomic status. Most societies are stratified or hierarchicalized in some way, where those who possess more power and economic resources are best equipped to both alter the stress-inducing situation and to ward off the harmful consequences of the stress. In the United States, women, ethnic and racial minorities, and those with fewer economic resources historically have held less power, been exposed more directly to health-depleting stressors, and possessed fewer resources for coping relative to their more advantaged counterparts. Today, however, studies find that each group has its own distinctive sources of strength and challenge as they manage stress.

Older and Wiser? The Impact of Age

We might think that when problems strike, they would exact a more harmful toll on older adults than on younger persons, because aging is associated with natural (albeit gradual) declines in physical vigor, strength, and mental sharpness. For some, old age is also linked to a shrinking social support system, as one's peers die or become too sick to provide support. Yet mounting research shows that older adults may be less susceptible than younger people to some of the physical and psychological blows that accompany stress. First, older adults are less likely to turn to unhealthy behaviors as a coping strategy. Persons in their sixties and older don't drown their sorrows in sweets and other unhealthy comfort foods because their dulled senses of smell and taste make eating less satisfying. Likewise, an older adult who has never smoked cigarettes or drunk alcohol will not likely hit the bottle or light up a Marlboro for the first time, whereas a younger person may take up bad habits anew when hit with a rough patch.

Second, the ups and downs of life are less emotionally devastating to mature adults than to younger persons. Older adults have lived through it all—deaths, divorces, wars, floods, and recessions. As such, they have years of experience coping with stress, and possess the knowledge that they can survive (almost) anything, and the emotional equanimity that comes with having done and seen it all. They're also less likely to be surprised by major stressors; while a younger person may be shocked and devastated by the unexpected death of a spouse, most older adults have at least some expectation that their spouse will die in the not-too-distant future. Some also rely on the advice and support of peers who have gone through similar losses.

Emotional reactivity also changes with age. As we grow older, we develop a greater capacity to manage or "regulate" our emotions, meaning that the highs are never as euphoric as those experienced during our heady teen years, but the lows are never as bleak. Older adults report less extreme levels of both positive and negative mood, and shorter-lived mood dips when a major negative event strikes. This more balanced emotional response to life's rhythms has both biological and social components, including decreases in autonomic arousal, adherence to cultural expectations that the elderly should not be "too emotional," and the attainment of wisdom, which may help older adults to respond to major stressors and daily nuisances with acceptance and perspective.

Yet older adults are not immune to the physical and mental health decrements that accompany stress. They are more likely than younger people to experience stress "pile-ups," or the accumulation of difficulties that can weaken our immune systems and threaten our cardiovascular systems. Older adults are more likely than younger persons to experience cognitive and physical declines, financial strains, multiple deaths of friends and loved ones, and the loss of important social roles, such as worker, spouse, and sibling. Age-related physical declines such as mild cognitive impairment, muscle weakness, fading vision and hearing, and sleep troubles may make them all the more susceptible to the health-depleting effects of stress.

A Weaker Sex? Gender, Stress, and Health

Men and women react to stress in different ways. In general, women are more likely to become depressed, whereas men are more likely to turn to drinking or even aggressive behavior when stressed out. Women also are slightly more likely than men to rely on emotion-focused than problem-focused coping, although this partly reflects social context and is changing rapidly over time. In past decades, women often lacked the financial resources to tackle some problems head-on, and instead might have turned to rumination, but these gender differences have attenuated over time. Studies consistently show that men and women adopt coping tactics that are consistent with gender-typed expectations regarding emotional display. Men are more likely than women to use PFC, control their emotions, accept the stress-inducing problem, not think about the situation, or show emotional inhibition or a "bottling up" of emotions. Women, by contrast, tend to seek social support, and use EFC tactics such as distracting themselves, releasing their feelings (e.g., crying or talking it out), or turning to prayer.

Yet is there a "weaker sex" when it comes to stress reactivity? The simple answer is no. No evidence shows that either men or women uniformly deal with stress less capably than the other; rather, each responds differently. Early writings suggested that women were more vulnerable to stress, yet these studies were often focused on female-typed responses to stress only (i.e., depression rather than aggression), or they failed to consider that women had fewer economic resources than men to resolve their problems. It's not surprising that a stressful event such as divorce would be more devastating to women than to men, especially in the mid-twentieth century. The word "divorcee" was whispered behind closed doors, revealing how shameful divorce was for women. Likewise, a woman who married young, had children, and lacked marketable career skills would be understandably distressed if she were forced to provide financially for her children postdivorce.

Current studies, by contrast, show that neither men nor women fare systematically worse in the face of divorce, yet the sources of their distress differ. Women still face some financial troubles and work-family strain following divorce, which compromises their sense of control and heightens feelings of depression. Men, by contrast, lose an important source of emotional support and social control, and may self-medicate their emotional pain by drinking. In sum, there is little evidence that there is an innate "his" and "hers" approach to stress and coping; rather, gender differences reflect larger social forces such as access to economic resources and socialization processes that "teach" men and women to respond to stress with very different emotions.

Minority Stress: Race and Ethnicity

Surprisingly little research explores racial and ethnic differences in responses to stress. This partly reflects the fact that there is wide within-group variation in how whites, blacks, Latinos, and Asians cope with stress. In other words, there is no "white" or "black" way of managing stress. The majority of studies explore the complex ways that race and social class intertwine, given that blacks and Latinos tend to hold fewer economic resources than whites and Asians in the United States. Most studies concur that ethnic minorities are more likely than whites to be exposed to stress, and that they also face an entirely separate set of stressors from which whites are spared. This "minority stress," as psychiatric epidemiologist Ilan Meyer calls it, includes exposure to race-based discrimination, prejudice, tokenism, and struggles to balance one's own cultural practices with those of the majority white society. These stressors, along with socioeconomic-status-based stressors, such as economic strain, dangerous neighborhoods, limited access to high-quality health care, heightened risk of divorce, and network events (such as children's imprisonment or unemployment), conspire to put blacks in particular at a heightened risk of developing health problems.

Given this onslaught of stressors, some blacks and Latinos may cope by turning to high-fat comfort foods and alcohol, which further increase their risk of illness, especially cardiovascular disease and diabetes. Epidemiologist Sherman James also observed a harmful coping style in African Americans that he dubbed "John Henryism." Named after the American folklore hero who worked himself to death while building a railroad tunnel, John Henryism refers to the process whereby some blacks expend very high levels of effort to succeed against all odds and to "prove themselves" in a majority white society. Unfortunately, this coping tactic exacts a physical toll. James and his colleagues found that blacks with high scores on John Henryism scales have an elevated risk of symptoms including high blood pressure. Just as John Henry died clutching his hammer, some African Americans may slowly suffer by working tirelessly to succeed in untenable and high-pressure situations.

However, Meyer and others argue that ethnic minorities also possess distinctive coping resources that help them to overcome stress and deflect some of the health assaults that accompany stress. For instance, African Americans may benefit from resources such as support from their religious community, protective religious beliefs, and high self-esteem. A strong sense of racial identity also protects against stress, especially racial discrimination. Ethnic pride, strong ties to one's ethnic community, and a sense of commitment to one's ethnic group protect against psychological distress in the face of discrimination. However,

public policies to eradicate race-based discrimination may ultimately enhance African Americans' health more effectively than
would an intervention geared toward enhancing ethnic pride.

Money Can Buy Health and Happiness: Socioeconomic Status

Socioeconomic status (SES), or one's level of education,
occupation, income level, and the assets one possesses is one of
the most powerful influences on our lives. As noted earlier, those
with fewer economic resources face a litany of stressors from
which their wealthier counterparts are spared, and they also lack
the economic and political resources necessary to change the
stressful situation. It's difficult, if not impossible, to move away
from a poor crime-plagued neighborhood if you don't have the
money for a downpayment on a new apartment. Quitting a miserable job isn't an option for those living paycheck to paycheck.
Those with little education may lack the cognitive flexibility to
devise creative solutions to their problems, nor have they learned
how to wrangle the social resources needed to fix a pressing
problem. Although people who lack economic resources may
have deep and emotionally rewarding social relationships, members of those social networks may be overburdened by requests
for help and support. As sociologists Leonard Pearlin and Carmi
Schooler have observed, "The groups most exposed to hardship
are also the least equipped to deal with it."

This unrelenting stress, combined with a dearth of coping resources, has direct effects on physical health, and leads to
sustained activation of stress-related autonomic and neuroen-
docrine responses, which leads to weakened immune systems.
Low SES also exacerbates the health consequences of a stressor,
whereas high SES minimizes these consequences. For example,
a team of researchers at the University of Michigan examined
whether middle-aged smokers who suffered a heart attack would
be more likely to quit smoking, relative to their counterparts
who did not suffer the stress of a heart attack. They found clear

evidence that a heart attack triggered smoking cessation, yet this effect was considerably larger for highly educated smokers. More highly educated persons have a deeper understanding of the link between smoking and heart disease, a greater sense of control over their environment, and a stronger belief that they can effect healthy change through their own behaviors.

Despite the overwhelming evidence that those with fewer SES resources fare poorly in the face of stress, studies still show great variety in how poorer people cope. A series of fascinating studies by Iowa State researcher Carolyn Cutrona found that living in a poor, dangerous neighborhood that lacked basic amenities such as good grocery stores and high-quality health care facilities is linked to depression. However, residents possessing personality traits associated with effective coping are far less likely to be depressed, despite their persistent neighborhood strain. For example, women with low levels of neuroticism, high levels of optimism, and a strong sense of personal efficacy were relatively immune to the depressing effects of neighborhood disorder. Taken together, these studies show how powerfully SES affects our lives, yet they also underscore that no single risk factor predetermines our health and well-being.

Lean On Me: Social Support as Source of Strength

If stress researchers were asked to name the single most important factor that distinguishes those who break versus those who merely bend in the face of adversity, most would immediately say "social support." Hundreds of studies document the importance of social ties as a resource that helps to ward off the health-depleting effects of stress. A core component is emotional support, such as having a confidante to listen to our problems, and feeling that our family and friends love, support, and listen to us in our times of need. Just as important, though, is instrumental and informational support. This refers to the practical support we receive when we're down. Instrumental support may include a loan so that a financially strapped friend can make her rent payment, or offering to babysit when an overwhelmed parent needs a break from their demanding children. Informational support includes recommending a good lawyer to a coworker going through a divorce, or sharing information within a sibling who is looking for a new job.

The benefits of social support are not limited to our mood and coping skills; it carries direct and indirect implications for our physical health as well. Close friends, family members, and significant others encourage their loved ones to engage in healthy behaviors (and kick bad habits) in the face of stress, helping them to forestall illness and infection. Close emotional ties also provide direct physiological benefits. As we saw in chapter 3, oxytocin is a chemical released when we have comforting physical contact with a significant other, whether a hug from a friend or satisfying sexual relations with one's partner. The release of oxytocin, in turn, has a protective effect that counterbalances the health-harming effects of other stress hormones.

It's no surprise that having loved ones who support us through thick and thin protects against stress-related health threats. But can short-term or fleeting support also help us to survive stress? The evidence is mixed, but generally yields the answer "no." One study by researchers at UCLA brought subjects into a laboratory and had them deliver a five-minute speech followed by a five-minute mental arithmetic test (i.e., the Trier Social Stress Test, described in chapter 3). Before engaging in the two stressful activities, the subjects were administered a small skin wound, so that researchers could investigate how quickly subjects healed. One half of the subjects were assigned a companion to help them with their speech. The subjects were told that the companion was available to help and to talk, if they wanted to. They also received support, advice, and words of encouragement from this companion when they were done with their tasks. The other half of subjects were not offered this support. The social support intervention had no effect on wound healing, blood pressure, or other physiological indicators. However, studies using a similar experimental design that had real-life spouses or best friends (rather than a research confederate) provide support to the research subjects do show a positive effect on health outcomes. Thus, social support is most protective when it's received in the context of long-term, high-quality relationships.

Yet can there be situations in which social support dampens our ability to bounce back from stress, perhaps by rendering us helpless or dependent? A handful of studies provides some evidence for this notion. Social support can heighten one's distress if the help provided is not what the recipient needs, if the recipient is distressed by the lack of reciprocity in his or her relationship, or if the support is delivered in a condescending or ham-fisted way. One study, aptly titled "The Way to Console May Depend on the Goal," shows that support needs to be consistent with the recipient's needs in order for it to be helpful. If the recipient feels guilty or indebted, then the support might even intensify the recipient's distress level. In sum, social support is protective if it's delivered in a way that is sensitive to the needs of the recipient.

Orchids and Dandelions: The Role of Genetics

Genetics play an important role in our hair and eye color, how easily we gain or lose weight, our risks of illness, and even our personalities. When centenarians talk about their long life spans (or supermodels explain their slender physiques or high cheekbones), they often thank their "good genes." Genes alone do not shape our destinies. Rather, our genes interact with the social situations we find ourselves in, and these combined forces have powerful effects on our physical and mental health. In recent years, researchers have identified specific genes that make us more or less susceptible to the harmful effects of stress. Researchers have developed a framework called the diathesis-stress model, which views some people as carrying genetic traits (called risk alleles) that make some wilt in the face of stress, while others blossom.

The model proposes that some people carry a gene that renders them highly sensitive to social and environmental factors. Those who are most vulnerable to negative social factors also benefit most from protective factors or positive events. These context-sensitive people have been referred to as "orchids." Just as an orchid needs the proper sunlight, water, and loving care to thrive, these context-sensitive people may blossom most successfully when provided with supports, such as encouragement, a positive childrearing environment, or a strong role model. The dark side is that they may be emotionally devastated by a stressor, such as childhood abuse or parental death. By contrast, "dandelions" are people whose behaviors and feelings are not highly affected by social environment. Although they may be saddened or depleted by a stressful situation, their reactions will not be as severe as that of the orchids. By the same token, they are also less amenable to the potential healing powers of resources like social support.

What makes someone a "dandelion" versus an "orchid"? Researchers have identified several genetic factors that amplify the effects of stress on health and well-being. The serotonin transporter gene (also known as SERT or 5-HTTLPR), has a particular variant (i.e., the "short" variant) that is implicated in depression and anxiety disorders. Another gene, DRD4-7R, is a variant of a dopamine-processing gene called DRD4 and is linked to several self-destructive behaviors, including conduct disorder, drinking, bullying, aggression, and sexual promiscuity. Advocates of gene-environment perspectives hold that if a person has a particular genetic vulnerability, he or she may respond all the more strongly to a particular stressor. The stress of law school may drive any student to drink, but the risk is even greater for students with the DRD4-7R gene. Likewise, a bad breakup may make us all sad and despondent, but the risk of major depression is even higher for those with the short SERT allele.

Research on gene-environment interactions is still in its nascent stages, but mounting evidence based on both survey data and lab studies finds that genes shape our stress responses. For example, one laboratory study at Stanford University found that teenage girls with the 5-HTTLPR allele experienced much higher levels of the stress hormone cortisol than did girls without the allele, following the completion of a stressful arithmetic task. Similarly, a large survey based on five hundred twins found that persons with the "short" allele variant of the 5-HTTLPR gene reported higher levels of depression in the face of stressful life events, relative to their counterparts without the allele. These studies are provocative, yet most scholars interpret these results cautiously. There are so many variants of our genes that scientists are certain to find a few that are linked to stress reactivity in some contexts and some studies. But will this particular risk allele be linked to reactivity in other contexts?

Others critics worry that the current scholarly emphasis on genes will lead some to throw up their hands and just assume that ill health and depression are predetermined for those who are born with a particular genetic predisposition. The narrow emphasis on genetic vulnerabilities may also detract attention from social vulnerabilities—such as poverty and lack of social support. The jury is still out, but evidence suggests that neither the biological nor social nor psychological alone is sufficient to help us understand stress responses. Although there is strong evidence that economic resources, social support, adherence to problem- rather than emotion-focused coping strategies, and possessing protective personality traits such as optimism or conscientiousness help buffer the health effects of stress, none of these resources singlehandedly explains all the variance in health or well-being in contemporary U.S. society. Our answers are best found by considering the complex array of factors that make our lives full. The proposed solutions to both stress exposure and reactions, highlighted in chapter 5, recognize that there is never a single bullet—biological or social—that accounts for the stress-health link. We now turn to some of those solutions.

CHAPTER 5

Paths to Healing

STRATEGIES FOR OVERCOMING LIFE'S STRESSORS

IT'S IMPOSSIBLE TO TURN on the television or pick up a magazine without seeing some new tips to battle stress. The past two decades have seen an explosion of popular books, magazine articles, and websites focused on reducing stress, but which tips work? And do particular strategies work better for some people than others? In this chapter, I briefly highlight those interventions, practices, or programs that have been identified as being effective for battling stress and its related health woes. Yet I also show that individual efforts to reduce stress (or to stay healthy in the face of stress) are only one part of the solution. Certainly, steps such as improving one's diet, talking to a therapist, doing deep-breathing exercises, changing potentially self-destructive thought processes, reaching out to friends and family, and, in some cases, relying on medications to reduce depression or anxiety are effective ways to survive a stressful time. Yet many of the stressors we face are not just personal problems; they're sweeping social concerns. Unemployment, lack of access to affordable childcare, difficulties in making an appointment to see a health care provider, the high costs of college, workplace discrimination, and widespread social pressures to "have it all" contribute to the stress levels of millions of Americans. Public policies to remedy problems such as poverty and limited access to health care may also be effective in helping us to battle stress and its consequences.

As we search for ways to minimize stress and its accompanying health effects, it's important to remember that stress affects people in different ways. As discussed earlier in the book, we know that our responses to stress vary based on our personalities, our ways of coping, how optimistic or pessimistic we are, the social support we receive, how much money and power we have to enact changes in our lives, and even our genetic makeup. We also know that different people experience different symptoms in the face of stress; some become depressed, some anxious, some angry. Some toss and turn all night and suffer from health-depleting sleep problems. Others take on unhealthy behaviors such as smoking, drinking, drug use, or "stress eating," each of which may give rise to health problems such as obesity, metabolic syndrome, diabetes, and high blood pressure. Our reactions are not due solely to personal traits or personal choices but are also linked to the nature of the stress we're experiencing, including its intensity, duration, and the accumulation of other related stressors. Understanding why, how, and for whom stress affects health is a critical first step in figuring out appropriate solutions. I'll briefly summarize a few of the most common strategies used to combat stress, and will show whether, how, and for whom they're effective.

CHANGING OUR BEHAVIORS

Our health behaviors are a critical pathway linking stress to health. Smoking, drinking, consuming copious amounts of caffeine, eating unhealthy comfort foods, and using illegal drugs might make us feel better in the short term, but each of these quick-fix mood enhancers may give rise to even more stress, health troubles, and anxiety. Yet kicking bad habits is easier said than done. Nicotine, drugs, alcohol, and even caffeine have addictive properties, which makes it hard for us to give them up. Most Americans who try to lose weight fail; scientific studies show that crash diets and weight loss drugs are ineffective. Weight Watchers is one of the few programs that has demonstrated long-term effects on weight loss. A study published in the international health journal *The Lancet* attributed the success of Weight Watchers to its social support component; the frequent "check-ins" and team-based approach boosted participants' motivation. This lesson applies to other health behaviors as well; those hoping to kick an unhealthy habit may find it's easier to do if they have friends also striving toward the same goal, or if they have regular "check-ins" with the friends and family members who care about them.

Kicking bad habits is just one half of the equation, however. The other is adding positive health behaviors, including giving oneself an extra hour of sleep each night, fitting in exercise at least three times each week, and cutting unhealthy foods from our diet and replacing them with healthy foods. Given that time pressures are a leading source of stress, experts advise that busy stressed-out people incorporate healthy behaviors into their regular daily routines. Taking stairs rather than the elevator at work, and walking rather than driving to nearby appointments is a quick way to add fitness to one's day. Ensuring that one's refrigerator is empty of sweets and fatty foods helps some to avoid these treats altogether. Adding fruits and vegetables to one's diet, even preprepared frozen produce, is a healthy alternative to fast food. Drinking water rather than coffee, tea, or cola not only calms down our nerves but helps us to sleep better at night and also fights the health-depleting symptoms of dehydration. Experts acknowledge, however, that it is impossible to make major behavioral changes overnight, and attempts to do so may increase our stress levels further by making us feel like failures. Slow and steady is the key. And few people can "get healthy" on their own; a supportive social network is essential.

Another important step toward reducing stress is cutting out of our lives those minor stressors we have some control over. As with healthy behaviors, this is easier said than done. At the very least, experts suggest that we try to find some balance between positive and negative experiences each day. Cancel a coffee date with a "toxic" or mean-spirited coworker, and instead schedule a friendly walk with a person whose company you enjoy. To the extent that it is possible, don't procrastinate. The distressing feeling of chasing an overdue deadline will then be replaced by a positive feeling of having completed one's task in a timely manner. Give yourself an extra ten minutes to commute from Point A to Point B; the stress of time pressure will be replaced with a few moments of replenishing downtime. Although many of us cannot alter the major stressors in our lives, we can make minor behavioral changes on a daily basis that may bring down our heart rates and enhance our moods a bit.

CHANGING OUR THOUGHTS

Can we "think" ourselves out of a stressful situation? The short answer is sometimes. As described in chapter 4, many effective coping strategies involve rethinking the stress in our lives. Strategies such as seeing the humor in a bad situation, finding meaning or benefit in a major challenge, or positively reframing a situation are associated with better mental health. By contrast, ruminating and catastrophizing are thought processes that increase our distress levels, and may actually lead to more stress. Ruminating, as discussed earlier, is the process whereby we dwell on negative aspects of our lives, including our mistakes. Catastrophizing is a thought process whereby we irrationally believe that a minor problem is far bigger than it actually is, often imagining a spiraling-out of negative consequences. For instance, a catastrophizer might get a speeding ticket, and then worry that taking a day out of work to contest the ticket will lead to lost pay and potentially being fired. But not taking the day out of work to challenge the ticket might lead to going to jail! Certainly, these imaginary thoughts could be highly distressing. Neurotic personality types are particularly susceptible to these harmful thoughts. By noticing when we engage in these harmful thoughts and then shifting our thoughts to more realistic or positive possibilities, we can minimize our emotional distress. For those who cannot shift their thinking on their own, receiving professional cognitive behavioral therapy (CBT) could be useful.

Some experts also call for greater spirituality in our lives; the belief that there is some "higher power" may help people to gain perspective, whereas others find solace in the belief that their current difficulties are quite minor and fleeting, in the grand scheme of things. Devotees of meditation swear that it helps to calm their minds and bring down their stress levels. Even those who are scared off by words like "meditation" could benefit by finding a few minutes each day to sit in silence, breathe deeply, and focus on a single image. This helps our minds to become less scattered, and adds focus and a sense of calm to our hectic lives. One particular blend of cognitive and spiritual approaches, mindfulness-based therapy, has been found to be particularly effective in fighting depressive symptoms, anxiety, and even psychosocial adjustment among cancer patients.

Although mental exercises like these might make us feel better in the short term, they are emotion-focused coping strategies that don't cut to the core of the stressor. Often, our situations must change if we want our stress to disappear. One of the most effective ways to cut down on worries and distressing thoughts is to streamline or cut back on one's obligations. As a recent Gallup Poll found, one of the most common sources of stress in the United States is the persistent feeling of time pressure. Experts suggest that we "just say no" when we're asked to take on another task that might put us over the edge stress-wise. Politely turning down invitations gives us more time to work on the tasks at hand, and helps our schedules to remain (relatively) uncluttered. Moreover, saying "no" to an opportunity—whether work or social—may lead to that opportunity being passed along to another person who may want or benefit from it more. For instance, turning down the invitation to serve on an important committee may give a junior colleague the opportunity to shine in the role. By "paying forward" a potentially rewarding opportunity, we might also bring ourselves a short-term mood boost.

REACH OUT TO A FRIEND

Social support is one of the most important resources we have for coping with stress. Our friends and family can provide a listening ear or a shoulder to cry on. Equally important, though, they may provide the practical support we need—whether a ride to a job interview, a cash loan to help pay bills, or a place to crash if our own home and spouse are the source of our stress. Many stressed-out people fear reaching out, however, because they think this signals that they're not capable of managing on their own. Yet this view is wrong-headed. One of the foundations upon which social relationships are based is reciprocity, or the assumption that in the future we will help out those who helped us in the past. Asking for help isn't a sign of dependence but rather the first step in what may be a long journey of "give and take" with loved ones.

Of course, not all people have a network they can reach out to. As noted in chapter 4, the people who face the greatest stress may also be embedded in social networks in which friends and family also are overwhelmed by life's challenges. In such cases, reaching beyond one's family and friends—perhaps to a local social worker or to a support group—may provide the assistance one needs. Although some people may be reluctant to reach out to strangers, thinking that "they'll never understand," one of the most effective sources of help is peer support, or peer counseling. Widow to Widow, for instance, is a long-running program that helps recently bereaved spouses to take care of themselves, manage their grief, and get their lives back on track. Recently bereaved persons are matched with a long-bereaved person who can serve as their mentor and guide them as they navigate their new role of widow. Psychotherapist Phyllis Silverman developed this program in the 1960s, and it has been a model for other peer-to-peer support systems. Peers understand what we're going through, and may provide not only thoughtful advice but also the assurance that it is possible to live through something as traumatic as widowhood and still find happiness and fulfillment in the future.

WHEN IS PROFESSIONAL SUPPORT NECESSARY?

When stress levels get too high, it may be desirable to see a professional, whether a clinical psychologist, psychotherapist, clinical social worker, psychiatrist, or general practice physician with whom one feels comfortable. These professionals are trained to help individuals, couples, and families to work through their stress, with many specializing in particular types of problems, ranging from marital troubles to eating disorders to major depression. Of course, not all people are comfortable seeking professional help. Studies have documented generational differences, in which older adults are reluctant to seek therapy for fear of the stigma that comes from needing help. Likewise, some ethnic and racial groups are reluctant to "air their dirty laundry" outside the confines of their homes and families. Still others find the cost of professional help to be prohibitive. Only very recently have most major medical insurances provided mental health benefits that are on par with physical health benefits. The Mental Health Parity and Addiction Equity Act of 2008 now requires that mental and physical health care coverage be roughly comparable.

Professional psychological help isn't the only kind of help we need in times of stress. Given the toll that stress takes on our bodies, it is essential that we seek timely and regular medical care to help detect early signs of trouble—such as high blood pressure, early onset of diabetes, or a high body weight that puts us at risk for other diseases. As with mental health care, high-quality medical care may be beyond the financial grasp of poor and uninsured Americans. Ironically, these are precisely the people who are most susceptible to stress and its unhealthy consequences. However, disparities in access to coverage changed in January 2014. Under the Affordable Care Act (ACA), all Americans now have access to many free services, including depression screening, substance use disorder screening, blood pressure screening, obesity counseling and screening, assistance with quitting smoking, vaccines against several infectious diseases, and counseling for domestic abuse victims. These services may help some to extricate themselves from stressful situations, such as abusive marriages, while they may alert others to the fact that their bodies and minds are succumbing to stress as evidenced by the results of depression and blood pressure screens. Although this health information alone cannot help all Americans, especially not those with limited access to health care, it is a first step toward detection and treatment for stress-related health conditions and symptoms.

MEDICATIONS

The number of Americans relying on medications to help them through times of stress has skyrocketed in recent years. An estimated one in ten Americans today is on antidepressants, and as many as one in four women in their forties and fifties rely on these medications. Most antidepressants fall into a class of drugs called SSRIs (selective serotonin reuptake inhibitors). These medications work by altering the naturally occurring chemical messengers (neurotransmitters) that communicate between brain cells. SSRIs block the reabsorption or "reuptake" of the neurotransmitter serotonin in the brain. Changing the balance of serotonin helps our brain cells to send and receive chemical messages, which in turn elevates our mood.

Although antidepressants are widely prescribed, they are not effective for everyone. Most mental health researchers have found that these medications are best suited for treating people with major depressive disorder (MDD), described in chapter 2. For people suffering from persistent and serious symptoms of major depression, medications can make a tremendous and positive difference. However, for people with mild depressive symptoms or sadness, these medications are far less effective. According to sociologist and mental health scholar Allan Horwitz, sadness is a "normal" response to many of life's stressors, such as divorce, death, or personal disappointment. Talking through the problem with a trained therapist or counselor, figuring out ways to move beyond (or change) the problem, and even the simple passage of time may be more effective than SSRIs for those experiencing such sadness. Talk therapy may not be equally effective for all, however. Its effectiveness may hinge on finding a good "match" and on persisting with therapy. One recent study by *Consumer Reports* found that therapy was most effective if patients stuck with it for thirteen visits. Although studies vary in what they deem the "magic number" of sessions one should attend, most agree that one visit is not adequate.

Changing Our Society

Social critics reading this chapter might be thinking that therapy, medication, and maintaining a healthy lifestyle are effective ways to cure the consequences of stress, but not the roots of stress itself. This would be an accurate appraisal. Many, if not most, of the stressors discussed in this book have their roots in major social inequalities based on one's social class, race, gender, age, or even body size. As such, we might hope for the enactment of public policies that could erode the main sources of stress in our lives. Let's revisit several of the people introduced earlier in this book, to show how social policies and interventions could have improved their lives. Recall Rob, the unemployed repairman, who committed suicide by gunshot after two unsuccessful years of searching for a job. Economic programs to enhance job training or increase job creation could have reduced Rob's stress regarding unemployment. Stricter gun laws might have stopped Rob from purchasing the very gun he used to kill himself. A culture that encouraged men to share their feelings of distress and disappointment rather than keeping their feelings of shame and anger bottled up might have given Rob the outlet he needed.

Now let's consider Marisol, the college student who exhausted herself while trying to carry a demanding course load and work full time. Expanded grant and loan programs for college students could have given her some reprieve from her daunting schedule. With a bit more sleep and less stress, her immune system might not have faltered and led to a bad case of the flu.

Naomi, our overburdened caregiver who had a stroke just months after her ailing husband and mother died, could have benefited from public programs to provide caregiving assistance. Public health insurance programs, such as those included in the ACA, might have enabled Naomi to get a timely doctor's checkup. Recall that Naomi had lost her insurance when her ailing husband took a disability leave from his job.

No one would argue that public policies are a cure-all. Nor are they sufficient to eradicate all sources of stress and stress-related health woes. By the same token, individual-level initiatives to live healthy lives and "think ourselves" happy also are not sufficient to eradicate stress and its consequences for our minds and bodies. Stress is a persistent part of life, and that fact will never change. In fact, some minor stress is good for us. It toughens us up, helps us to develop coping skills, and keeps us "on edge" just enough that we force ourselves to prepare for the stressful tasks we foresee in our future. Yet persistent and accumulated stress can have long-term and devastating effects on our life spans and daily well-being. Public policies, individual behaviors, and community efforts to support one another in times of need, together, may be the most effective way to ensure that all Americans can lead lives marked by health, happiness, and peace of mind.

Recommended Reading

Chapter 1 Introduction: What Is Stress?

American Psychological Association. (2012). Stress in America: Our health at risk. Washington, D.C.: APA. Retrieved from http://www.apa.org/news/press/releases/stress/2011/final-2011.pdf

Becker, D. (2013). *One nation under stress: Social uses of the stress concept.* New York: Oxford University Press.

George, L. K. (1999). Life-course perspectives on mental health. In C. Aneshensel & J. Phelan (Eds.), *Handbook of the Sociology of Mental Health* (pp. 565–583). New York: Kluwer.

Holmes, T. H., & Rahe, R. H. (1967). The social readjustment rating scale. *Journal of Psychosomatic Research, 11,* 213–218.

Pearlin, L. I., Lieberman, M. A., Menaghan, E. G., & Mullan, J. T. (1981). The stress process. *Journal of Health and Social Behavior, 22,* 337–356.

Pearlin, L. I., Schieman, S., Fazio, E. M., & Meersman, S. C. (2005). Stress, health, and the life course: Some conceptual perspectives. *Journal of Health and Social Behavior, 46,* 205–219.

Rosenquist, J. N., Fowler, J. H., & Christakis, N. A. (2011). Social network determinants of depression. *Molecular Psychiatry, 16,* 273–281.

Selye, H. (1956). *The stress of life.* New York: McGraw-Hill.

Sorensen, M., et al. (2012, June). Road traffic noise and incident myocardial infarction: A prospective cohort study. *PLoS One.* Retrieved from http://www.plosone.org/article/fetchObject.action?uri=info%3Adoi%2F10.1371%2Fjournal.pone.0039283&representation=PDF.

Thoits, P. A. (1995). Stress, coping, and social support processes: Where are we? What next? *Journal of Health and Social Behavior* (Extra Issue), 53–79.

Wheaton, B. (1990). Life transitions, role histories, and mental health. *American Sociological Review, 55,* 209–223.

CHAPTER 2   SWEATING THE SMALL (AND BIG) STUFF:
HOW AND WHY STRESS AFFECTS OUR MENTAL HEALTH

Almeida, D. M., McGonagle, K., & King, H. A. (2009). Assessing daily stress processes in social surveys by combining stressor exposure and salivary cortisol. *Biodemography and Social Biology, 55*(2), 219–237.

Archer, J. (1999). *The nature of grief: The evolution and psychology of reactions to loss.* Routledge: New York.

Centers for Disease Control. (2013). Suicide among adults aged 35–64 years—United States, 1999–2010. *Morbidity and Mortality Weekly Report* (May 3, 2013).

Heatherington, E. Mavis, & Kelly, J. 2002. *For better or for worse: Divorce reconsidered.* New York: Norton.

Higgins, E. T. (1987). Self-discrepancy: A theory relating self and affect. *Psychological Review, 94,* 319–340.

Horwitz, A. (2009). Mental health, adulthood. In D. Carr (Ed.), *Encyclopedia of the life course and human development* (pp. 279–288). Farmington Hills, MI: Cengage.

Kessler, R. C. (2010). The prevalence of mental illness. In T. L. Scheid and T. N. Brown (Eds.), *A handbook for the study of mental health: Social contexts, theories, and systems,* 2nd ed. (pp. 46–63). New York: Cambridge University Press.

Meyer, I. H. (1995). Minority stress and mental health in gay men. *Journal of Health and Social Behavior, 36,* 38–56.

National Institute of Mental Health. (2012). *Bipolar disorder.* Washington, D.C.: NIMH. Retrieved from http://www.nimh.nih.gov/health/publications/bipolar-disorder/nimh-bipolar-adults.pdf.

Radloff, L. S. (1977). The CES-D scale: A self-report depression scale for research in the general population. *Applied Psychological Measurement, 1,* 385–401.

Schieman, S. (2006). Anger. In J. E. Stets & J. H. Turner (Eds.), *Handbook of the sociology of emotions* (pp. 493–515). New York: Springer.

Seery, M. D., Holman, E. A., & Silver, R. C. (2010). Whatever does not kill us: Cumulative lifetime adversity, vulnerability, and resilience. *Journal of Personality and Social Psychology, 99*(6), 1025–1041.

Tedeschi, R. G., & Calhoun, L. G. (2004). Posttraumatic growth: Conceptual foundations and empirical evidence. *Psychological Inquiry, 15,* 1–18.

Wallerstein, J., Lewis, J. M., & Blakeslee, S. (2001). *The unexpected legacy of divorce: A 25 years landmark study.* New York: Hyperion.

Yerkes, R.M., & Dodson, J. D. (1908). The relation of strength of stimulus to rapidity of habit-formation. *Journal of Comparative Neurology and Psychology, 18,* 459–482.

CHAPTER 3 UNDER OUR SKIN: HOW AND WHY STRESS AFFECTS OUR PHYSICAL HEALTH

Cohen, S. (2004). Social relationships and health. *American Psychologist, 59,* 676–684

Detweiler-Bedell, J., Friedman, M. A., Leventhal, H. E., Leventhal, E., & Miller, I. W. (2008). Integrating co-morbid depression and chronic physical disease management: Identifying and resolving failures in self-regulation. *Clinical Psychology Review, 28,* 1426–1446.

Dimsdale, J. E. (2008). Psychological stress and cardiovascular disease. *Journal of the American College of Cardiology, 51,* 1237–1246.

Galea, S., Tracy, M., Hoggatt, K. J., DiMaggio, C., & Karpati, A. (2011). Estimated deaths attributable to social factors in the United States. *American Journal of Public Health, 101,* 1456–1465.

Jordan, J. (Ed.), Bardé, B. (Ed.), Zeiher, & Andrea, M. (Ed.) (2007). *Contributions toward evidence-based psychocardiology: A systematic review of the literature.* Washington, D.C.: American Psychological Association.

Kiecolt-Glaser, J. K., & Glaser, R. (1994). Caregivers, mental health, and immune function. In E. Light, G. Niederehe, & B. Lebowitz (Eds.). *Stress effects on family caregivers of Alzheimer's patients* (pp. 66-74). New York: Springer Publishing.

Phelan, J.C., Link, B.G., & Tehranifar, P. (2010). Social conditions as fundamental causes of health inequalities: Theory, evidence, and policy implications. *Journal of Health and Social Behavior,* 51, S28–S40.

Martikainen, P., & Valkonen, T. (1996). Mortality after the death of a spouse: Rates and causes of death in a large Finnish cohort. *American Journal of Public Health, 86,* 1087–1093. Retrieved from http://www.apa.org/monitor/feb08/oxytocin.aspx.

McEwen, B. (2002). *The end of stress as we know it.* New York: Dana Press.

Reczek, C., Pudrovska, T., Carr, D., & Umberson, D. (201). Marital status, marital transitions, and alcohol use: A mixed-methods study. Annual meetings of the American Sociological Association.

Sapolsky, R. (1998). *Why zebras don't get ulcers: An updated guide to stress, stress-related disease, and coping.* New York: Freeman.

Segerstrom, S. C., & Miller, G. E. (2004). Psychological stress and the human immune system: A meta-analytic study of 30 years of inquiry. *Psychological Bulletin 130* (4), 601–630.

Umberson, D., Crosnoe, R., & Reczek, C. (2010). Social relationships and health behavior across the life course. *Annual Review of Sociology, 36,* 139–157.

Chapter 4   Why Some Crumble and Others Bounce Back: Risk and Resilience in the Face of Stress

Carver, C. S. (1997). You want to measure coping but your protocol's too long: Consider the Brief COPE. *International Journal of Behavioral Medicine, 4,* 92–100.

Carver, C. S., & Connor-Smith, J. (2009). Personality and coping. *Annual Review of Psychology, 61,* 679–704.

Connor-Smith, J. K., & Flachsbart, C. (2007). Relations between personality and coping: A meta-analysis. *Journal of Personality and Social Psychology, 93,* 1080–1107.

Cutrona, C. E., Wallace, G., & Wesner, K. A. (2006). Neighborhood characteristics and depression: An examination of stress processes. *Current Directions in Psychological Science, 15,* 188–192.

Dobbs, D. (2009, December 1). The science of success. *The Atlantic Monthly.* Retrieved from http://www.theatlantic.com/magazine/archive/2009/12/the-science-of-success/307761/.

Ehrenreich, B. (2009). *Bright-sided: How positive thinking is undermining America.* New York: Picador.

Gotlib, I. H., Joormann, J., Hallmayer, J., & Minor, K. L. (2008). Biological stress reactivity mediates the relation between genotype and risk for depression. *Biological Psychiatry, 63,* 847–851.

James, S. A. (1994). John Henryism and the health of African Americans. *Culture, Medicine, and Psychiatry, 18,* 163–182.

Kendler, K. S., Kuhn, J. W., Vittum, J., Prescott, C. A., & Riley, B. (2005). The interaction of stressful life events and a serotonin transporter polymorphism in the prediction of episodes of major depression. *Archives of General Psychiatry, 62,* 529–535.

Lazarus, R. S., & Folkman, S. (1984). *Stress, appraisal, and coping.* New York: Springer.

Nolen-Hoeksema, S. (2004). *Women who think too much: How to break free of overthinking and reclaim your life.* New York: Holt.

Pearlin, L. I., & Schooler, C. (1978). The structure of coping. *Journal of Health and Social Behavior, 19,* 2–21.

Shepperd, J. A., Klein, W. M. P., Waters, E. A., & Weinstein, N. D. (2013). Taking stock of unrealistic optimism. *Perspectives on Psychological Science, 8,* 395–411.

Zoccola, P. M., & Dickerson, S. S. (2012). Assessing the relationship between rumination and cortisol: A review. *Journal of Psychosomatic Research, 73,* 1–9.

CHAPTER 5   PATHS TO HEALING: STRATEGIES
FOR OVERCOMING LIFE'S STRESSORS

Fourner, J. C., et al. (2010). Antidepressant drug effects and depression severity: A patient-level meta-analysis. *Journal of American Medical Association, 303,* 47–53.

Hofmann, S. G., Sawyer, A. T., Witt, A. A., & Oh, D. (2010). The effect of mindfulness-based therapy on anxiety and depression: A meta-analytic review. *Journal of Consulting and Clinical Psychology, 78,* 169–183.

Horwitz, A., & Wakefield, J. (2007). *The loss of sadness: How psychiatry transformed normal misery into depressive disorder.* New York: Oxford University Press.

Jebb, S. A., et al. (2011). Primary care referral to a commercial provider for weight loss treatment versus standard care: A randomised controlled trial. *The Lancet, 378,* 1485–1492.

Silverman, P. R. (2004). *Widow to widow: How the bereaved help one another* (Series in Death, Dying, and Bereavement). New York: Routledge.

Singletary, M. (2013, September 17). Mental-health coverage to get a big boost under Obamacare. *Washington Post.* Retrieved from http://articles.washingtonpost.com/2013-09-17/business/42146528_1_essential-health-benefits-preventive-services-mental-health-coverage.

About the Author

Deborah Carr is a professor in the Department of Sociology and Institute for Health, Health Care Policy, and Aging Research at Rutgers University. She has published widely on the ways that work and family stress affect health. She is the author or editor of several books, including *Spousal Bereavement in Later Life* (2006) and the *Encyclopedia of the Life Course and Human Development* (2009).